# A CONSULTATION WITH THE
# **BACK**DOCTOR

# A CONSULTATION WITH THE
# **BACK**DOCTOR

DR. HAMILTON HALL, M.D., FRCSC

M&S

*To Peter,*
*thank you*

**National Library of Canada Cataloguing in Publication**

Hall, Hamilton, 1938-
A consultation with the back doctor / Hamilton Hall.

Includes index.
ISBN 0-7710-3778-3

1. Back – Care and hygiene.  2. Backache.  I. Title.

RD768.H356 2003      617.5'6      C2002-905701-9

We acknowledge the financial support of the Government of Canada through the
Book Publishing Industry Development Program and that of the Government of Ontario
through the Ontario Media Development Corporation's Ontario Book Initiative.
We further acknowledge the support of the Canada Council for the Arts and the
Ontario Arts Council for our publishing program.

Published simultaneously in the United States of America by McClelland & Stewart Ltd.,
P.O. Box 1030, Plattsburg, New York 12901

Library of Congress Control Number: 2002116597

Typeset in Minion by M&S, Toronto
Printed and bound in Canada

This book is printed on acid-free paper that is
100% ancient forest friendly (100% post-consumer recycled).

This book is not intended to replace the services of a physician.
Any application of the recommendations set forth in the following pages
is at the reader's discretion and sole risk.

McClelland & Stewart Ltd.
*The Canadian Publishers*
481 University Avenue
Toronto, Ontario
M5G 2E9
www.mcclelland.com

1  2  3  4  5      07  06  05  04  03

# Contents

# PREFACE

It has been a quarter-century since *The Back Doctor* was published. I realize how much has changed every time I look at my face on the cover of that book. This was a time long before the fall of the Berlin Wall, before e-mail and the Internet changed the way we communicate, when *Jaws* terrified us and Kojak's lollipop kept us entertained.

Back then, the goals of *The Back Doctor* and *More Advice From the Back Doctor* seemed radical. Advocating activity instead of bedrest, independent knowledge instead of reliance on a health professional, and a simple, commonsense approach to managing back pain were strange concepts. My lectures to professional and lay audiences were met with scepticism and even a tinge of hostility.

How things have changed! Today, prolonged bedrest has been shown to be not only ineffective, but also potentially harmful. Sufferers are deluged with information and self-help advice. Shark cartilage and eponymous exercise routines have challenged the primacy of the medical practitioner. Surely, with all this progress, back pain will soon be a thing of the past, as remote from our daily lives as diphtheria or the Black Death.

There has been so much progress, and yet so little has changed. Back and neck pain have not disappeared, and the toll in human suffering and economic disruption continues to rise. Back pain is the leading cause of lost workdays and is second only to coughs and colds as a medical reason to visit the doctor. Neck pain afflicts over half those who already suffer problems in the low back. What's wrong? Why do we seem unable to reap the rewards of decades of research?

This book will try to give you some of the answers. Over the past years, the problem of spinal pain has not been simplified or even adequately explained. Increasing technological complexity, which permits investigations, treatments, and surgeries that were beyond our reach a generation ago, has often led to greater confusion, unrealistic expectations, and a steady increase in the number and expense of both useful and useless therapies. Clearly, differentiating between what helps and what doesn't can be extraordinarily difficult.

Back and neck pain are conditions prone to frequent, prolonged periods of spontaneous remission. No matter how severe, every acute attack will end. Except for an unfortunate few, predominantly those caught in the web of pain-focused behaviour, periods of pain are interspersed with periods of relative comfort. Although the recurrence rate is high (over 50 per cent within two years), each individual episode typically diminishes or disappears within three or four months. Improvement can occur within a few weeks, and sometimes within a matter of days. Not surprisingly, treatments with no legitimate value often claim credit for recoveries that might have happened anyway. This makes it difficult for the sufferer to know whether it was the treatment or the passage of time that brought relief. And this difficulty is greatly worsened when the therapy that appeared to produce relief was purchased at considerable personal expense. Could anyone admit to being so gullible as to spend significant amounts of money to produce an effect that would have occurred by itself? It is so much easier and safer for the ego to believe the therapy works.

The elusive promise of technology is reflected in the growing number of alternative non-surgical treatments for neck and back pain. For example, traction during bedrest, long since discredited as having any lasting effect, has been replaced by traction applied with the aid of a computer. The delivery system comprised of a flat surface, ropes, and straps is essentially the same, and so is the result. Why would an identical treatment augmented with meaningless high-tech information produce a consistently superior result? It doesn't. But where traction in bed required only a pelvic belt, a length of rope, and a sandbag, computer traction requires a hundred-thousand-dollar machine to generate a series of treatments that can cost the patient several thousand dollars.

Spine surgery, an approach often wrongly viewed as the last resort, does have a place in treating some clearly defined mechanical problems. Back or neck surgery done by the right surgeon on the right patient for the right reasons carries a success rate in excess of 90 per cent. Unfortunately, choosing the correct operation for the correct patient is still difficult – in some circumstances, virtually impossible. In spite of our ability to image the spine, the surgeon may still be unable to isolate the specific pain source. Even where the point of pain is identified, there may not be any chance of a successful operative intervention. Regrettably, this does not always lead to a refusal of surgery. An unnecessarily desperate patient and an inappropriately confident surgeon are a dangerous combination.

The flood of information available over the Internet and echoed in the popular press is vast, detailed, and largely inaccurate. Repeated analyses by professional organizations suggest that more than half of this information is misleading. A greater problem in obtaining useful information is that, for neck and back pain, remedies that work for some do not necessarily work for others. There is no universal solution.

Thirty years as an orthopaedic spine surgeon has changed my perspective. The original *Back Doctor* offered advice on postures, exercises, and even bedrest that I no longer recommend. Yet over the years, I have had hundreds of patients tell me that the advice in that book helped them overcome their pain and return to normal activity. Did I help them by providing the wrong information? I don't think so. I believe the benefit of *The Back Doctor* lay primarily in its descriptions of the problems we all face in trying to get information about a frightening subject from professionals who don't fully understand the terrifying impact of their casual comments. *The Back Doctor* stressed the importance of understanding the benign nature of back pain: that although the specific source of pain cannot be identified, the underlying problems are easily understood, and, in most cases, readily controlled. I have come to believe that a specific exercise or activity is less important than the attitude that directs it.

When I wrote *More Advice From the Back Doctor* eight years later, I incorporated a number of back-extension exercises and positions for pain control. This expansion of my approach was due largely to the influence of Robin McKenzie, a physiotherapist from New Zealand. Robin and I share many beliefs about the management of neck and low back pain, particularly the importance of self-directed care and the need for practical patient education. Robin was also the first to describe the phenomenon of centralization, a shift in the location of back and neck pain that serves as a guide in evaluating the effectiveness of mechanical therapy.

During my early attempts to develop patient education materials, I realized that without establishing a specific pathology or cause, back and neck pain could be classified according to the symptoms. By combining what the doctor sees (the signs) with what the patient feels (the symptoms), it is possible to create a picture of back pain that can be recognized by most sufferers. Having your personal affliction identified and illustrated is a great comfort to many people. Knowing that your problem is not unique and that many others have successfully overcome the same pain eliminates a lot of uncertainty. You are not alone in your struggle.

My original concept described three types of pain, each associated with a specific underlying physical problem. I later added a fourth type and then, to the consternation of many of my patients and colleagues, I reversed the order of the first two types.

A great step forward for this pain classification, now called "patterns of pain," occurred when it became the basis for neck- and back-pain management within the Canadian Back Institute (CBI). In 1974, I had begun a series of informal patient-education lectures designed to provide the basic information and practical skills needed to control simple mechanical pain.

From that modest beginning, CBI expanded first as a multi-centred educational program, and then, in the mid-1980s, as a series of active treatment centres. The program to control mechanical neck and back pain was gradually extended to include the treatment of a variety of musculoskeletal complaints and chronic pain. Today, CBI operates over one hundred and twenty locations across Canada, some in affiliation with regional hospitals or local sports clubs, and some as separate facilities. The CBI has locations in Hong Kong, Brazil, and New Zealand. Its staff are active in workplace ergonomics and in assisting return to work. Now called CBI Health, the program has expanded far beyond its original parameters and has developed a complete business structure, an active research and publication section, and one of the largest coordinated databases on neck and back pain in the world.

But although its focus and interests are now wide-ranging, the core of the CBI approach is still the patterns of pain. The introduction of these patterns into a clinical setting required that they become both immutable and resilient. Using nothing more than the clinical presentation, the patterns must provide sufficient clarity to permit both useful discussion among clinicians and the development of appropriate treatment plans. The original types and the early patterns were not equal to the task. Over many years and through numerous meetings and consultations, the patterns were strengthened and simplified to meet these difficult demands. The work of dozens of skilled and experienced clinicians has created the patterns as they exist today and as they are described in this book. My special thanks to Maureen Hunt, Tony Melles, Rob Stewart, Greg McIntosh, Christina Boyle, Rob Karas, Chris Szybbo, and Tom Carter for their invaluable contributions. They and many others have converted my recognition of the particular characteristics of neck and back pain into a powerful clinical tool.

Surprisingly, I discovered that the value of the patterns increased as their link to any specific pathology weakened. Although it is natural to wonder why the pain exists, the more immediate concern for most patients is, "How can I make my pain stop?" These pain patterns are based on the clinical picture: the signs and symptoms provided by the patient and supported by the clinician's findings. No specific organic cause is required to establish the pattern. The identified pattern then directs the individual's initial treatment routine for rapid pain control. If the patient's history corresponds with the physical examination, and if both these in turn are confirmed by the predicted elimination of symptoms and return to function, then the pattern is both established and verified. Of greater importance, the patient's major concern, elimination of pain, has been addressed. Treatment is empirical: if it works, it must be right. The theories of causation are secondary. Each pattern has its putative pain source, and I will discuss these, but the important issue and the strength of the approach is that pattern recognition offers a safe and reliable method of initiating prompt relief. It is an approach that transforms an ominous but vague threat into a simple and finite solution.

Perhaps the final answer for our lack of progress in conquering neck and back pain is its extensive, unfortunate, and unnecessary medicalization. For over seventy years, the medical profession has worked to turn neck and back pain from an unfortunate human condition into an illness. It has created a disease for which it has no cure. A disease, moreover, that need not exist. By suggesting that the problem can be eliminated, medical science has raised expectations to an unrealistic level. Neck and back pain are not about to disappear. They will never be extinguished as long as humans live and grow old. No drug, treatment, or surgery offers a panacea. Yet the pain of a sore neck or a sore back can be controlled and, in most cases, abolished, at least for a time.

This book is my attempt to provide each reader with a personal consultation; a chance to ask and receive answers to the questions about your back and neck pain that have troubled you. It is an opportunity to offer to a wider public the practical advice I dispense every day in my clinic. I have chosen to use the question-and-answer format that I employed in *More Advice From the Back Doctor*. It seems particularly suitable for the task at hand.

Chapter 16, "On the Ball," is based on *Ball Bearings*, written by Jeff Compton, Stefan Scott, and Matt Tyler. Jeff and Stefan are kinesiologists and Matt is a physiotherapist. If you are looking for additional information about using the exercise ball, I heartily recommend their book.

I appreciate the assistance I received from Professor John Edmeads in preparing Chapter 6, "This Thing Gives Me a Headache." Dr. Edmeads is Canada's foremost expert on headaches. I value his opinion, and it was gratifying to see a neurologist and an orthopaedic surgeon in such close agreement.

It is a pleasure to work again with my two favourite illustrators, Professor Margot B. Mackay and Mr. Peter Honor. Both have added immeasurably to my publications. Jonathan Webb and the editorial staff at McClelland & Stewart were invaluable. My special thanks goes to Adam Levin for his "merciless" review of the manuscript.

I am particularly indebted to Dr. Susan Grant Hall, my general medical consultant, in-house editor, and wife.

The information in this book represents the state of our art today, and some of it will, in the years ahead, be surpassed by newer technology. What will not change, and what has remained constant since I began my practice, is my belief that back and neck pain are best managed by their owner, and that, outside the operating room, my most important contribution is to offer information, guidance, and support. I cannot assume responsibility for someone else's recovery. I can offer genuine encouragement that the problem can be mastered.

# CHAPTER ONE

---

## *Why Am I Here?*

I suspect that this classic question is in the mind of many of the patients I see every day in my office. I know it is a question I frequently ask myself as I listen to their stories of back and neck pain. We view the same frustration from very different perspectives. For most patients, I am the second, third, or tenth professional they have consulted about their problem. They cannot help but ask themselves what good one more consultation can do and what advice they can possibly expect to be given that has not been followed unsuccessfully before. From my perspective, I despair that so many patients have received so much misinformation or useless recommendations. I am disappointed that so many have been given an extensive course of therapy, exotic programs of obscure exercises, or even a recommendation for surgery, but have never been provided with the basic information about the causes and elementary mechanical control of back and neck pain.

If the question is not already in the patient's mind before the consultation, I'm sure it arises the moment I begin to discuss simple strategies to decrease pain by improving the way they sit or lie in bed at night. Having seen so many other practitioners, and having waited so long, the patient expects my consultation to include a little magic, a minor miracle, or, at the very least, some new and technologically advanced equipment. One way or another, the expectation is the same, as is the response to my offered advice. "I haven't waited this long/come this far/seen so many others just to sit here listening to simple common sense."

But that is what back- and neck-pain management is all about. Until it was turned into a medical condition in the early twentieth century, back pain was considered an inevitable human experience. It still is. There is no simple cure because there is no obvious illness. Over 90 per cent of people who suffer neck and back pain suffer the effects of normal ageing and the inevitable results of daily activity on the structures of the spine. Just like hips and knees, backs will eventually wear out.

At this point, there is nothing that medical science or alternative therapies can do to prevent the inevitable. Age, or "advanced maturity," as I prefer to call it, is a fact of life.

So is neck and back pain. Research indicates that about two out of every three people who experience pain in the spine cannot identify any specific event as a cause of their problem. In the majority of cases, back pain just happens. It happens in spite of the use of a proper ergonomic chair, a change in the work schedule to minimize long periods of sitting or standing, the use of mechanical aides for lifting or materials handling, and even diligent attention to a back-exercise program. It is a sad truth that back pain, like advanced maturity, cannot be prevented.

But it can be controlled. In most cases, that control begins with understanding the problem, and with recognizing that the basic responsibility to care for your back and neck rests with you.

You have a choice. You can allow your back to rule your life by letting it influence your every decision, however big or small. Falling into that trap leads to a life of chronic pain and a pattern of self-destructive behaviour. Your alternative is to devise a strategy for taking charge, so that *you*, not your neck or back pain, will determine how you live and what you do with your life.

Once you have resolved to take control, the trick is to pursue your strategy with single-minded determination without letting it become an obsession. Your focus must remain on the things that you do, and not on whether it hurts to do them. Constantly reminding yourself and others that you are struggling against the presence of pain is not the answer. Normal people don't act as if they have back pain. Normal people behave normally. That is your goal.

My message that simple actions and common sense can defeat your back and neck pain is not as popular as you might think. Many people just want to offload the problem to someone else. I sometimes think they come intending to leave their pain with me in the clinic and go home symptom-free. From my perspective, I often question my own reason for being here when I realize that the help I will provide is not the help the patient is looking for.

### Scenario #1
**I've had back pain for six months, but my doctor can't find anything wrong. Can't you order a CT scan or an MRI (or better yet, both of them) to find the trouble?**
It always comes as a surprise to patients to learn that the source of mechanical back pain cannot be located with an X-ray, computer tomography, or magnetic resonance imaging. These techniques can be used to identify the rare case of disease affecting the spine or to provide the exact location for a surgical approach, but they are of no value in the routine assessment of ordinary neck and back pain. Unfortunately, the promise of technology has raised expectations, and many patients will not be satisfied until a picture is taken.

There are three reasons I generally decline this request. First, the information will offer me no assistance. Second, it is an unjustified expense in a health-care system that is already financially strained. And third, all three types of studies are likely to show me signs of ageing, a narrowed space between the bones, a bulging disc, or a small bony spur that may not be present in the young, healthy spine. All of these are expected in an older spine, and are probably unrelated to the patient's current problem. Reporting these findings, however, usually increases the patient's concern rather than providing reassurance.

When the patient's focus is narrowly restricted to obtaining imaging studies and their request both understandable and inappropriate, there is little I can do.

## Scenario #2
**Twenty years ago, I slipped in the warehouse and twisted my back. Last month it started to hurt. Compensation has refused my claim. Will you help me and fill out my forms?**

A claim for compensation, disability, or insurance coverage requires proof of a specific event. Since most back pain just happens, and since all of us have in the course of our lives suffered incidents that are capable of injuring the spine, there must be direct and recent relationship between the time of the accident and the onset of the pain to have them related as cause and effect. The sequence must make sense. Back and neck pain are not illogical.

Furthermore, compensation insurance and disability decisions are administrative, based only in part upon objective medical evidence. As much as many people believe otherwise, the doctor is not the final arbiter in these situations. My goal is to offer assistance in the management of a physical problem, not to fulfil clerical requirements.

## Scenario #3
**My neck pain is awful. What can *you* do to make the pain stop?**

Probably nothing. Purely passive treatment (therapies provided by someone else without the sufferer's participation) rarely have any enduring effect. Massage, adjustment, cold-pack application, or prescription medication can produce short-term benefit, but by themselves they offer little hope of lasting improvement. In this scenario, even if I do offer immediate help, the patient's approach of asking what *I* can do portends a poor result. Back and neck pain can be managed; I have already made that point. But they require the active participation of the owner. Waiting for someone else to solve the problem is not the answer. People travel great distances and spend considerable amounts of money seeking the solution only to find, like Dorothy in *The Wizard of Oz*, that the answer is right in their own backyard.

## Scenario #4
**My doctor says I need an operation on my back. When can you perform the surgery?**

Probably no more than two people in a hundred will benefit from spine surgery. It is definitely not the answer to controlling simple mechanical back and neck pain. The decision for surgery is not based only on how much it hurts. Successful spine surgery depends upon two things: the ability to clearly identify the source of pain and the fact that removing, immobilizing, or replacing that pain source will eliminate the symptoms. Surgery cannot resolve pain-driven behaviour, reverse the generalized effects of ageing, restore total loss of function within the spinal cord, or repair fully established nerve injury.

The decision for surgery should be taken by the operating surgeon in conjunction with a well-informed patient. While it is not a treatment of last resort, and should not be delayed unnecessarily, neither is it a judgement to be made in haste or without full knowledge of all the circumstances.

Sadly, in some cases, a patient's enthusiasm to accept early surgery is more an indication of his or her willingness to relinquish responsibility than the outcome of a carefully calculated decision on the merits of an operation.

Like most spine surgeons, I am cautious about accepting another physician's evaluation that a patient needs an operation. I am particularly cautious when that opinion comes from one of my non-surgical colleagues. Doctors as well as patients tend to overrate the value of surgery, or at least to extend its positive influence far outside realistic limits. Surgery does have its place, and in its place it can be strikingly successful. However, as a surgeon facing a patient who does not require surgery but who will entertain no other option, I find myself in a corner: what I have to say won't be heard.

## Scenario #5
**I've had back pain on and off for the last ten years. I've seen my family doctor many times and he has sent me to a number of different specialists, who've given me a lot of advice. One even thought I needed an operation. I tried to learn more about my**

**condition on the Internet but I got confused. I'm looking for some answers about why I hurt and what I can do to make the pain go away. Can you help?**

In this scenario, I know why I am here. Providing specific advice on neck and back care requires that I first determine the nature of the problem, establish the characteristics of the attack or attacks, and attempt to classify them into one of the four basic patterns of mechanical pain. Once I have made that judgement I will be able to recommend specific postures, pain-control activities, and exercises that can both diminish the present pain and defend against future recurrences.

# CHAPTER TWO

## *Start with the Basics*

I believe it is easier to develop an effective pain-management routine and establish lasting mastery over your back and neck symptoms if you base your approach on your particular pattern of pain. But before I address the specific problems of each pattern, there is a lot of general information every sufferer of back and neck pain should know. A range of activities can be easily modified to reduce discomfort. Every victory builds confidence and that, in turn, builds a positive attitude. Success depends on the knowledge that you are not in danger of doing yourself harm and the belief that you are capable of overcoming the pain. Without the proper perspective you may be beaten before you begin.

I can think of two patients whose different attitudes illustrate the profound effect of your approach. One patient, a woman in her late forties, had been coming to me for years with a chronic back problem. She was originally an active woman but had developed a lifestyle that increasingly focused on her pain. She would highlight her suffering, for example, by requesting a wheelchair whenever she travelled through an airport. Although her physical condition was stable, her attitude continued to deteriorate. I remember asking her at one point how she was coping.

"I am not," she said. "I have given up everything, even grocery shopping. I can't lift those heavy bags."

I asked her why she couldn't have someone else carry her groceries to her car or pack them in smaller bags and make more frequent trips.

She replied, "Even if they took them to the car at the store I would still have to carry them into the house when I got home. And I haven't got the time to go back and forth with more bags."

Since she had already given up everything else, I was puzzled as to what she planned to use the time for, but I chose not to ask. This patient had become good at rejecting any positive suggestions that might help resolve her problem. Despite my many attempts to provide her with reassurance and constructive advice, she remained determined to dwell on her pain and to defy anyone to help her get better. There is little that I can do or say when a patient refuses to be helped.

In contrast, there was the twenty-three-year-old man I saw some years after he had fractured three bones in his spine in a diving accident. Contrary to popular belief, not all spinal fractures result in permanent disability. In this case, the outcome was normal function despite an obvious deformity in the middle of his back, marking the point where the bones had been crushed. Initially, the pain was intense, but over time, as it does with other fractures in the body, the pain diminished. He began an intensive back-strengthening program, and by the time I saw him, his pain was under control. He experienced some occasional discomfort, but no more than most people would consider normal.

The patient's problem was not his back injury or back pain, but the fact that he could not get a job. With limited education and no trade experience, the only work available to him required heavy physical labour. All his prospective employers had turned him down because of his back. In spite of the fact that he was now capable of normal activity, he still felt compelled to report his accident. What was even more frustrating to me was the fact that his doctor supported his continued restrictions. He had undoubtedly sustained significant trauma and had been left with the visible evidence of a healed spinal fracture, but there was no longer any reason for physical limitations or need for continued caution. The patient was not even experiencing any substantial pain. In short, there was no reason why he could not go back to work, any work.

I recommended that the next time he applied for a job he just tell them that he was ready to go rather than describe his prior injury.

"But don't I have a permanent problem?" he asked. "My doctor warned me that I would never be normal again."

"Don't you feel normal?" I asked. "Aren't you able to do the things you want to do?"

"Of course I am. But I was sure from what I have been told that it would be the wrong thing to do."

To ease his mind and to satisfy any future employer, I gave him a letter certifying that he was fit for all duty and sent him on his way. He got a job and shortly after that a promotion. He now considers his back injury a thing of the past, as it should be. It is the attitude we carry forward, not the pain we leave behind, that matters.

### Is back pain inevitable?

No, but it is very likely. Estimates of the frequency of neck and back pain in industrialized countries run between 60 and 80 per cent of the adult population. Although the majority of these episodes are short-lived, and most subside spontaneously, they do constitute a major problem. Although the pain cannot be prevented, it can certainly be managed through a variety of simple and self-directed routines.

### If I can manage the pain, why can't I just avoid it in the first place?

Most back pain doesn't come from a single physical injury. It is the result of the stresses and strains we all place on our spine during everyday activities. These inevitable minor insults, combined with the natural wear of advancing maturity, lead to back pain.

With time, the discs between the bones of the spine become less resilient and their surfaces may crack or bulge. The outer shell of the disc is pain-sensitive, and anything that disrupts the surface hurts. The small joints linking the bones together gradually lose their incredibly smooth surfaces.

They can become painful, just as you would expect from ageing in the hip or knee joints. Occasionally, these accumulated changes produce pressure in one of the local nerves, adding yet another potential source of pain.

In most cases, during the early years, none of these changes hurt. Then one day, a routine lift or a familiar posture may push things a little too far and the pain begins. The principle is the same as when a split appears at the knee in an old pair of jeans: although you did nothing different, the worn fabric finally reached a point where one more bend was all it took to make it tear.

Often, with the strong incentive of possible financial compensation, people can describe the exact moment and the precise activity that caused the pain to start. But in most cases, the pain comes as a complete surprise.

### And I suppose the worse the wear has been up to that moment, the more painful the first attack will be.

Oddly enough, that is not so. The amount of pain often bears little relation to the seriousness of the problem. We can suffer a lot of pain from a back condition that is nothing more than a minor sprain of a small joint. The surface of the disc has the same type of pain receptors as the surface of the eye, and a small disruption can cause big pain. You know how much it hurts when you have even a tiny piece of grit in your eye.

The opposite is also true. There are some conditions in the spine, such as sustained pressure on a nerve, which can produce an injury such as permanent muscle weakness with little or no pain.

### If back and neck pain is so common, what hope do I have?

The attacks may be inevitable, but their duration and intensity can be significantly reduced. Some attacks can be completely aborted by assuming a specific position or immediately carrying out a series of neck or back stretches. No one need just accept the pain, and certainly no one should quietly endure the associated loss of function. We all have the ability to fight back.

### So I need a strategy. Can you suggest a standard set of rules or guidelines?

Because no two people experience exactly the same pain, there is no one set of rules. One size does *not* fit all. The more we understand about the problem, the more we are able to offer individual programs for specific problems. That is one of the great benefits of the pattern-recognition system discussed later. There are, however, a number of general strategies that can be applied.

### So what are the general principles of good back and neck care?

The best-known set of guidelines was published nearly ten years ago by the U.S. Department of Health and Human Services, Agency for Health Care Policy and Research (AHCPR). The AHCPR guidelines pertain to acute low back pain in adults, but the advice applies equally to acute neck pain. The guidelines were an attempt to review all the available medical literature on the subject of back-pain management and then present a synopsis of the advice best supported by current research and understanding.

Although the report fills a small book, the guidelines can be summarized in a few lines.

- In the absence of any indicators of potentially serious underlying spinal disease, or of generalized illness that may be affecting the back, imaging studies such as CT or MRI, or other medical tests, are not necessary within the first month of the onset of back pain. This recommendation applies to each acute episode. To take an extreme position, someone whose back pain never lasts more than a week never needs to be investigated.
- Bedrest longer than four days is not helpful and may actually lead to further disability. This is particularly true in patients with back-dominant pain without evidence of nerve-root irritation. Although the small number of patients with leg-dominant nerve pain recover more slowly and may require longer periods of intermittent rest, they too can expect improvement, and require no additional early investigation.
- Pain relief can be accomplished most safely with non-prescription medication or spinal manipulation.

- Patients recovering from an acute attack are encouraged to return to work or their normal daily activities as soon as possible. Both low-impact aerobic activities and trunk-conditioning exercises can be resumed within a week or two.
- The guidelines emphasize that the overwhelming majority of back-pain sufferers, even those experiencing pain from a pinched nerve, will make a full and complete recovery. There is an extremely limited role for surgery.

Taken together, the AHCPR guidelines can be summarized like this: Stay active; don't stay in bed, rely on non-prescription medication, or simple mechanical therapy for pain relief; start exercising and return to your normal lifestyle as quickly as possible. Above all, be reassured that the condition is temporary, and that full recovery is the usual result. Allowing the pain to limit your life can cause more serious and longer-lasting problems than just working through the discomfort and going back to your regular activities.

**So, even though it hurts, using my neck or back is not a dangerous thing to do.**

Right! Pain can be a great disincentive to activity, but in most cases involving the spine, hurt is not the same as harm. Activity may hurt a little, or even a lot, because it may aggravate a sore disc, joint, or muscle, but it is highly unlikely to cause physical injury. When you feel pain, your back isn't necessarily saying, "This is damaging me." More likely it is saying, "You're making me do something I don't want to do. Are you sure you want to go ahead with this?" Your spine often asks the same question after a day digging in the garden or an hour hiking in the hills. The correct answer, if you need to get the job done or if you are enjoying the activity, is "Yes, I do. I am not going to do you any harm. Just stay with me until we are through."

There are many times when you may consider it worthwhile to ignore a pain message from your spine. There will also be occasions when you choose to avoid the pain because there is nothing to be gained by putting up with it. And there is a lot to be said for feeling comfortable. However, once you realize that the hurt does not signal a serious problem, you can make your decisions based upon the importance or the enjoyment of the activity. If it feels good, do it. If you want to do it but it hurts, do it anyway.

**But surely some things people do must be bad for their backs. I have heard so many stories about people who have injured themselves at work or after a lifetime of heavy lifting. Aren't some activities or occupations harder on the back than others?**

Of course, some things put more strain on the spine. And there are certain occupations, such as nursing or mining, where there is a well-accepted increase in the incidence of reported back and neck pain. But the picture is not as clear as you might expect. Do people in heavy jobs requiring repetitive bending and lifting have more back pain? Or does the nature of their job make the back pain they have more disabling? Surprisingly, research has never proven that heavy work injures the spine. Back pain is also well known to office workers. Neck pain in particular has become epidemic among people who work at a computer. The frequency of reported back and neck pain, and the degree to which they disrupt your life, will depend more on your ability to change the way you do your job and your desire to keep going than on any underlying physical insult.

I have had back pain most of my life but, except for a brief periods, it has never stopped me from doing the things that I enjoy or have to do. As a spine surgeon, I am required to stand for long periods bending over an operating table. The nature of the work makes it impossible for me to move very much or change my position. There are days when I find it a very uncomfortable thing to do but the work itself is sufficiently demanding that my back pain can be ignored until the operation is over and I can return to the surgeon's lounge and start complaining.

Consider a woman who works on an assembly line. She is required to bend forward and perform a light duty repeatedly during the day. Assume that the line is set up in such a way that she has no option as to how she must bend, and so the same activity is repeated over and over again. If she comes to work with a sore back, say, from spending too much time in the garden on the weekend, that back pain will be increased during her workday, and she will have no opportunity to avoid the discomfort.

Now consider another woman, who works in a job that requires her to perform essentially the same movements. Her activity level is as great, and through the day she will be required to bend as frequently as the woman on the line. But she can start and stop the activity as she wishes, speeding up to compensate for the times that she pauses to rest. And she has the opportunity to change her position, perhaps to work from the opposite side, or even to carry out her task perched on a high stool. The changes in timing and posture mean that even with a sore back she is much more likely to make it through her day with less pain than the assembly-line worker.

Another factor that has become increasingly important in our understanding of back- and neck-pain disability is the satisfaction that someone gains from his or her job. It is well-recognized that people who enjoy their work and feel they are making a significant contribution are more likely to continue, even with some back or neck discomfort, than are people who find their job unpleasant and dread the start of each workday.

The things that cause harm to the back are generally obvious, such as falling from a second-storey window or being hit by a pickup truck. Injuring your back by lifting a paper cup, bending over to tie your shoe, or sitting in a poorly designed desk chair are entirely different matters. Back pain is common, actual back injury is rare.

**From what you say, I don't think you will be giving me a list of things to avoid. But there are so many things I do every day that affect my back or neck. There must be some options that are better than others, aren't there?**

First, remember that, except for major injuries, there are very few things that you can do to physically harm your back. But there are a number of choices you can make during the day that will help your back and neck feel better. Certain lifestyle changes also offer an opportunity for long-term comfort and protection. I will talk about the long-term approach in Chapter 8, but first, let's look at some of the things you can do at any time to keep your back comfortable or to reduce the severity of a current attack.

Perhaps the most important principle is to keep moving. Back and neck pain can tighten the muscles along your spine so much that it seems impossible to move. Common sense would suggest that anything so painful should be kept very still. But I know from personal experience and from the comments of thousands of patients that the pain actually diminishes as movement returns. No doubt those first efforts will be very unpleasant, but keep reminding yourself that the hurt is not a sign of harm. Moving your back won't break it.

One of the best examples of this rule is a condition in the neck called torticollis, a long name that describes a sudden, spontaneous neck-muscle spasm (also known as "wryneck"). It occurs most often in children, adolescents, and young adults. The spasms strike for no particular reason and can last from a few days to a week or more. The muscles are tightest and most painful in the morning. They are sufficiently tight that the head is twisted to one side. Any attempt to turn in the opposite direction increases the pain. The natural response is to hold your head still and hope the neck pain goes away. The correct approach is to keep turning your neck against the spasm. At first you will not be able to move very much, but even a small gain helps. Don't try to force your head all the way to the other side. Pull gently and repeatedly against the tight muscles. Adding a little heat often lessens the pain and improves the movement. By the end of the day, you will have a significant increase in the range and a decrease in the pain. At night, without that constant stretching, the symptoms tend to return and morning will again be the most difficult time. But with continued stretching, each morning is better than the one before, until the spasm and pain disappear.

Torticollis is one specific example of the general principle. Painful muscle spasm tends to decrease if you can restore movement. Like that cramp in the calf of your leg that strikes during the night and sends you flying out of bed and hopping around the room, a sore neck or back needs to be moved.

This may seem a contradiction, and many of my patients never seem to make the connection. Yet they often tell me with some surprise that their back feels better after they have been active or exercised. It disturbs me when they then confide that the activity was done against the advice of their doctor, who had recommended strict rest. Despite the fact that their increased movement produced a positive result, patients are often concerned that they have done something wrong. In reality, if it feels good, it's good to do it.

**Is just feeling good a useful guide to choosing my activities?**
Generally, yes. Backs and necks are not injured in secret. If something makes your neck or back feel better, then it is probably the right thing for you to do. But that does not mean that everyone should do the same thing. For some, spending an hour working in the garden will leave their back feeling better than it has all day. For others, an hour of squatting and bending forward will be an hour of agony. The activity that brings you comfort will depend upon the pattern of pain that you experience, and I will be discussing those patterns in Chapter 3.

**But I have heard so much about choosing the right chair or mattress or car seat. Are you telling me that there is no perfect choice for everyone?**
Right again. There are a few general guides that can help you make your choice. As far as benefits to your neck or back are concerned, the cost of the item is not one of them.

Let's talk about chairs first. There is an old Monty Python sketch that includes torture in a "comfy" chair. The irony, I am sure unintended by the writers, is that most people's idea of a comfy chair – that large, soft, overstuffed piece of furniture – would be torture for many back- and neck-pain sufferers. The arms of the chair are often so high that you can't use them to help support your body. The seat is so deep from front to back that you can't rest your feet comfortably on the floor. And the back of the chair is so soft that it provides no support. Your back sags as you slump into it until your spine is curled forward like the letter C. For many people, staying in this position triggers back pain. And to compound matters, as your lower back slumps forward, your neck compensates by arching backward. Now you have the potential for neck pain as well.

A comfy chair looks comfortable and initially feels comfortable because it is soft. But the softer the chair, the less it is able to support your spine and the more it can contribute to your backache. I remember one man who convinced himself that the stress of his marriage was causing back pain. He would return from work feeling fine, but within a few hours of being at home with his wife, his back would start to hurt. I recommended that before he saw a marriage counsellor, he change the chair in his living room: the comfy chair where he sat for a couple of hours to read the newspaper. A new chair with better back support relieved his pain and saved his marriage. Because of all the discussion surrounding the new chair, his wife had the opportunity to suggest that he might better spend those first hours at home interacting with his family, anyway.

### For the sake of my back and my relationships, would I be better off sitting on a wooden kitchen chair?

Not necessarily. The slope of the back, the size of the seat, and whether or not the chair has arms all make a difference. Many kitchen chairs do not provide sufficient support for the low back and, although they are rigid, they don't hold you in the right position. When you think of all the furniture designed for so-called comfortable sitting, you can begin to appreciate the complexity of the problem.

Of course, not all seats are designed for comfort. Some are designed for convenience. The folding chairs in a community hall or school gym often have a metal bar across the top but no support at all for the lower back. They may be easy to stack but they make it difficult to stay comfortable during the children's recital. The hard, backless bench, the kind you see in many shopping malls, is another example of convenience over comfort. A bench offers no back support, and sitting slumped forward with your hands or elbows on your knees may feel comfortable for a few minutes but for most people that comfort won't last. If you stay that way too long, you'll find that your back feels sore when you straighten up. Maybe that's what the shopping-mall designers want: to make sure that you won't sit too long before you get up and start shopping again.

The Muskoka or Adirondack chair is another interesting example. These are the large wooden chairs seen outside everyone's cottage, with the markedly sloping seat and back and the wide wooden arms. Without added cushions, its comfort is short-lived, and if you have a sore back, getting out of that chair can be a challenge.

In fact, for people who find sitting uncomfortable, getting up from any chair can be a painful exercise. The same forward-bent position that brought on the problem in the first place is accentuated when you try to stand up. Your first move in leaving the chair is to flex forward. This puts your chest over your knees as you push up with your legs. You can avoid that sudden, unnecessary pain by sliding your buttocks to the front of the seat and then standing straight up without bending your back.

### I have heard about a chair where you kneel rather than sit. How does that work?

The seat of that chair slopes forward and most of your weight is taken through your knees on a padded knee rest. The kneeling position automatically puts a curve into the small of your back and that is a good position. But the design also puts a substantial load on your knees, and for some people that may not be pleasant. I wouldn't recommend buying a chair like that on the basis of its scientific theory. Even kneeling in it for a short time might not give you an adequate indication of its merit. I recommend that you personally test any unusual or expensive chair with as much actual use as you can arrange before you purchase one.

### What's the best chair for my back?

There is no such thing as the perfect chair. We are not all the same shape or size and we do not all have the same pattern of back or neck pain. A chair that suits one person may not suit another. A colleague of mine, a plastic surgeon, found it uncomfortable to perform surgery while sitting on a standard operating-room stool. He designed his own chair. It looked for all the world like a big, old-fashioned tractor seat. To him it was the ultimate in working comfort. And he wasn't alone. Whenever he was out of the operating room, several other surgeons used to compete for the pleasure of sitting in that seat. But not everyone found it comfortable.

I once visited the shop of a craftsman who specialized in custom-making chairs for maximum comfort. He used a simple system of heavy mesh screen and movable wooden rods to shape a chair exactly to the contours of your back and your backside. I was quite taken with his approach. He didn't try to impress me with a lot of scientific theory about the biomechanics of the spine; he just worked to make absolutely sure the result would suit the contours of the client's body. His whole approach was simply, "I will build whatever feels comfortable to you."

There are other high-tech solutions. Computers design chairs based on scientific theory. Seating contours can be created by having someone sit on a chair whose surface is a plastic bag filled with small beads. Once the beads have shifted to conform to the shape of the spine, the air within the bag is extracted and the compacted beads form a rigid mould. There are air-cushioned seats in the cabs of many long-haul trucks.

The rocking chair is a good example of how shifting body weight and spinal position while seated can bring prolonged comfort. A doctor friend of mine is part of a company that has developed a low back support for car and airplane seats that cycles through a slow process of inflating and deflating as you sit. This gradual change in support and position has proven to be effective. You might regard it as a high-tech rocking chair.

### Can you offer guidelines to someone looking for a good chair for an office job? Is an ergonomic chair the right choice?

There are a few general principles. Find a chair that supports the small of your back in its normal forward curve, the position doctors call lumbar lordosis. There should be a balance between excessive rigidity and too much "give." The back of the chair should tilt backward ten to twenty degrees, to suit your comfort and needs, and it should have a means of being locked into place at the angle you prefer. Some office chairs can become rocking chairs, and although that makes it difficult to type at your computer, it can certainly prolong your sitting comfort. Having the ability to switch between rigid sitting and rocking mode is a desirable feature.

Make sure the seat is deep enough to support the length of your thighs and wide enough to allow easy position change. If you are going to be seated for long periods, you will want to be able to switch from one side to another, to cross and uncross your legs, lean forward, lean back, and so on.

No matter how well-designed the chair may be, if you remain immobile for long stretches, you're inviting pain. The chair should have armrests that allow you to transfer some weight from your upper body to your arms and temporarily reduce the load on your lower spine.

Check the height of the chair seat against your desk or work surface to ensure that when you are seated with your arms at your sides and your forearms parallel to the floor, your work surface is at the level of your elbows. The back of the chair should be high enough to support your head and neck in a comfortable position, and that position should be level with your computer monitor. The chair should let you rest your feet easily on the floor to reduce the amount of weight taken by the backs of your thighs. And even with the best possible chair, you might do well to place a stool or a thick book on the floor in front of you so you can prop one foot up now and then. Or you might do what I do at my desk: pull out a low drawer and rest your foot on that.

Height adjustment is an excellent addition. You can raise or lower the chair to the seating height that seems exactly right for you and for the particular task at hand. It is a good idea to vary the height of your seating from time to time while you work. As for ergonomic chairs, an inexpensive sponge-filled lumbar roll in a simple wooden chair can provide adequate back support. The decision to use a particular piece of furniture should be based on the convenience and cost as well as the biomechanics. Good back and neck support is important, but you can be kind to your back and your budget at the same time. The right chair need not be the most expensive one.

No matter how good the chair, though, it is wise to stop work every half hour or so to get up and move around for a few minutes. Contrary to what the boss might think, the time out will not diminish your productivity but can, in fact, increase your output, since you won't spend the rest of your day distracted by your backache.

## Is there such a thing as the perfect way to sit?

For most of us, the best way to sit maintains the same normal contours of the spine that appear when you are standing erect. Try a simple experiment. Have someone observe you from the side as you sit casually in a typical living-room chair. Take particular note of the position of your head above your shoulders, using a point in front of your ear for reference. Now stand and face the same direction, and have your friend make the same observations. What the observer will notice is that when you stand, that point in front of your ear, and therefore your head, draws backward to balance more evenly on top of your shoulders. The head-forward sitting posture is a major contributor to neck pain, particularly for people who spend their days working at a desk or on a computer. Although most people don't realize it, changing the position of your head and neck when you sit can be easily accomplished by increasing the amount of curve in your lower back. The two curves, cervical lordosis in the neck and lumbar lordosis in the lower back, tend to balance each other. When most people stand, they increase the arch in their lower back and that is why they automatically improve the posture in their neck. A perfect way to sit mimics a perfect way to stand.

Most people are also surprised to learn that the load on the shock-absorbing discs in the spine is greater when you sit than when you stand up. That's why people with disc-related back pain would rather stand than sit.

### Sitting comfortably sounds like more of a challenge than I thought. What about sitting in the car?

Car seats have come a long way over the years. The old-fashioned bench seat has been greatly improved, and many of the new vehicles have switched to individually contoured seats. The luxury models feature multiple adjustments that allow you to change the tilt of the back and the seat as well as add a degree of lumbar support.

The principles we have already discussed still apply, but there are some additional factors. Most of these apply to the driver. Putting your feet on the pedals restricts the position of your legs. It means frequently lifting your feet off the mat, a movement that puts additional stress on the muscles in your low back. Gripping the steering wheel changes the position of your shoulders, and the stress of driving in heavy traffic or poor weather pushes your head forward as the muscle tension builds across your shoulders. Poorly placed headrests that shove your head too far forward can give everyone in the car a headache. It is little wonder that many people report back or neck pain after a long car trip.

My suggestions are similar to those we have already talked about. Additional low back support, in the form of a sponge roll, small pillow, or even a folded towel, can help. Positioning the support correctly requires some care and precision. I strongly recommend that you organize things before you start to drive, not while you are in traffic.

No matter how comfortable the seat, or how well you have placed your extra supports, driving for several hours is likely to produce neck and back discomfort. Stopping for a brief stretch every so often makes good sense. Changing your seat position, particularly the distance between the seat and the foot pedals, will change your posture. Adjusting the height of the steering wheel is another useful trick. On a long drive, you can spend time sitting like a bus driver, with the seat high and steering wheel up close and as high as possible. Some of the time you can drive with the seat lower and well back, and bring the steering wheel down, as if you were handling a racing car. Between these two extremes, there are numerous combinations that can change your posture and shift the point where you load your spine.

Seat belts are unquestionably a major advance in automobile safety. Although a seat belt reduces your freedom to move about, you can still shift your positions frequently. When applied properly and combined with adequate low back support, a seat belt can actually improve spinal posture.

## What about sitting on an airplane?
Although some improvements have been made in airplane seating, embarking on a long flight with a bad back can still be a daunting prospect. Airlines require that you keep your seat belt fastened at all times, and that obviously restricts your ability to move around. Being trapped in the middle of a three-seat row between two generously proportioned individuals, both of whom insist on using the armrests, is equally confining and socially more awkward to remedy. I have no surefire suggestions for that situation, but I can offer some useful in-flight tips.

First, always fold one of the small airline pillows into the small of your back to add additional lumbar support. Second, when you tighten your seat belt, tighten it low across your hips so that, just as in the automobile, the pillow and the belt will enhance your spinal posture. Third, put something under your foot so that you can use it as a footstool. As I have heard so often, "The aisles must be clear for takeoff and landing," but there is nothing to stop you from using a footrest during the remaining hours of your flight.

Finally, ask for an aisle seat so that you can stand up and move about several times during the trip. Although you may feel self-conscious lining up for the bathroom six times in seven hours, your back will thank you for the increased mobility. And a quick glance at the glazed expressions on the faces of your fellow travellers will confirm that they are not the least interested in your activities.

I know that you were asking me about seats on a commercial airliner. But your question brought to mind a recent experience I had flying in a small, four-seater aircraft. As part of a speaking trip to the Yukon, I had been invited to take an air tour of the ice fields. It was a spectacular flight, and one marred only by the fact that my back was killing me. I had just climbed into the seat next to the pilot and was still crouched down in the unfamiliar confines of the small cabin. The pilot reached over to help adjust my seat belt, which came over both of my shoulders as well as around my hips. To ensure that I would not be thrown about, should we experience any turbulent air, the pilot snugged the belt tight, forcing my shoulders down and firmly securing me in a flexed position. Rather than appear ungrateful, I said nothing, but by the time we were airborne, I sincerely wished I had. I was sufficiently unfamiliar with the mechanism of the belt that I chose not to try to adjust it myself, and by then the other two passengers were already admiring the view and the pilot was busy flying the plane. If I had ever had any doubt that sitting is harder on the back than standing up, or that being locked in a forward-bent position for two hours was a bad idea, that flight answered my question.

**If sitting is so hard on the back and I am too tired to stand up, what about lying down? If there is no perfect chair, does that mean there is no perfect mattress either?**

Like so many other elements of good back care, there are general principles and no firm rules. A good mattress is one that provides uniform support for the body, keeping the spine in as straight a line as possible.

Over the years, many people with sore backs have been told that it would be a good idea to sleep on the floor. Although I agree that a firm surface is generally more comfortable than one that is too soft, I think the floor is going a little too far. When you sleep on your side, as most of us do, the body is supported only at the shoulder and the hip. Without a pillow, the head falls to the side, and even with a pillow, the neck is unsupported. There is also no support for the spine below the ribcage and above the pelvis.

Mechanical back pain occurs when sensitive areas of the spine are subjected to long periods of load. Lying on your side with your neck and low back sagging like a clothesline between two poles places uneven pressure on many of the structures in your spine. That can lead to pain. Patients frequently tell me that their worst back or neck pain is in the morning, before they have the chance to get up and get moving.

### I often have backaches in the morning. Is it time for me to buy a new mattress?

Not necessarily. The position in which you sleep is often more important than the surface on which you sleep. Selecting the best sleeping position will depend on the pattern of your pain, and even then it is usually a question of trial and error. Waking with a sore back does not mean that you have harmed yourself overnight. There is no danger in experimenting with several new positions.

One of the best tricks I know is to use a rolled towel to support your neck or low back. Rolling a towel up and placing it inside the lower edge of your pillowcase will create a lump that fills the gap between your shoulder and your ear. Similarly, rolling up a couple of towels and laying them across the bed just above your waist will have the same effect on your lower back. In both cases, the diameter of the roll must be large enough to actually elevate the spine. And in both cases, this may mean that the roll is large enough to feel uncomfortable.

The question of comfort versus pain control is one that needs a few extra words. The purpose of using the towel at your neck or waist is to reduce or eliminate the typical pain you experience when you awake each morning, or which prevents you from going to sleep at night. The discomfort that comes from lying over the rolled towel is quite different from your typical pain, and it is important that you separate the two. The lump is uncomfortable because it is firm and it is placing your spine in an unfamiliar position. But this position can eliminate your typical pain. Patients are often told to avoid things that they find uncomfortable. As sensible as it sounds, in this situation, that is not good advice. Unless the roll under your neck or low back is large enough to change the position of your spine, it can't have any effect on your pain. A larger lump may be more uncomfortable, but if it is effective in stopping your usual pain, that discomfort will be a small price to pay. What is even better is that after you have used the roll for a few days, the new position becomes familiar and comfortable while the old pain stays away.

### I'm a restless sleeper, so how can I keep the rolled towel in the right place?

The towel rolled inside your pillowcase tends to stay where it belongs, but the roll at the waist can move as you shift in your sleep. If the towel under your low back won't stay put, you can try fastening it around your waist by wrapping the towels around a bathrobe sash and tying the sash around you. Even better, you can slide the rolled towel inside the leg of a pair of pantyhose and then tie the pantyhose around your waist. The roll must be large enough to change your posture so that when you fasten it around your middle, you should resemble the Michelin Man. I often tell patients that if the roll isn't large enough to make your partner laugh, it's not large enough to do any good.

### I've heard that a pillow between my knees helps. Is that true?

The pillow should be fairly bulky and it should be placed between your thighs, more above your knees than below. Having it between your legs maintains the alignment between your spine and your pelvis and causes you to roll over as a single block rather than twisting your hips first and then your shoulders. The pillow also limits how far you can turn onto your stomach. If reducing rotation in your spine and preventing stomach sleeping makes your back feel better, then a pillow between the knees is for you. You can certainly give it a try. It is a good experiment.

If your symptoms increase as you bend forward, sitting up to get out of bed can increase your back pain. One solution is to roll onto your side and then use your arm to push up. Keep your back straight and lower your legs over the side of the bed as you raise your upper body sideways.

### What about using a special pillow for my neck?
Most cervical pillows are designed with a ridge along the lower edge that fills the gap between your ear and your shoulder just as the rolled towel did. Whether you use the towel or a commercial pillow depends on comfort and cost. I have had success with a water pillow designed to create a bulge under my neck with the water displaced by the weight of my head. For me, it worked very well, but the first two people to whom I recommended the water pillow found it made their neck pain worse. Sometimes, you can't predict what will work.

### What about a waterbed or those new space-age materials that say they're recognized by NASA?
These alternatives offer good uniform support, and many people with neck and back pain find them helpful. By now you won't be surprised to hear that they don't work for everyone. Because of the nature of the support, you tend to move less frequently as you sleep, and therefore stay in one position for much of the time. For many people, sleeping this way provides pain control, but others find that maintaining any position for a long time increases the discomfort.

### What about a hammock?
There is something about the image of a warm summer afternoon, a cold drink, and a hammock rocking gently under the trees. It seems unfair to point out that the typical hammock prevents you from changing position

easily and tends to hold you in a slightly curved position without applying additional support to your neck or low back. I always enjoyed the image more than the reality, at least the reality after the first hour or so. But again, that is personal experience, and your experience may be different.

### What advice do you have about the best way to stand up?

There is less load on the discs of your back when you stand up than when you sit. Backs and necks usually feel better when they are moving. For both these reasons, many people with back pain find it more comfortable to stand and walk slowly than to sit or even lie down.

The goal is to balance the normal curves of your back: the lordosis, or forward curve, in the neck and low back, and the kyphosis, or backward curve, in the middle of your spine where the ribs are attached. Balancing these curves allows us to stand erect, and it spreads the load on the spine across the cushioning discs and the interlocking small joints as evenly as possible. The load-sharing effect is further improved as we walk around. As our weight shifts from side to side, different areas of the spine are briefly loaded and then allowed to relax. Since walking actually rotates the pelvis and produces a gentle twisting motion in the low back, it also helps stretch tight painful muscles.

### Someone told me that wearing high-heeled shoes or cowboy boots is bad for the back. Is that true?

It gets a bit repetitive, but each time I am asked a question like that, I first emphasize that these sorts of things are never bad for the back in a physical sense. They do not cause physical harm. The question should more properly be asked, "Do high-heeled shoes and cowboy boots cause back pain?"

The answer to that question is a definite "maybe." Elevating your heels increases the arch in your low back. For some patterns of back pain, increasing this arch is an excellent way to reduce the discomfort, and so wearing higher heels actually makes your back feel better. For others, increasing the arch is a certain way of increasing the pain. These people are more comfortable in flat-soled shoes. It is a question of comfort rather than a question of harm.

My pattern of back pain feels better with an increased back arch, and for many years I have worn cowboy boots even with a business suit. It drives the guy in the men's clothing store crazy. I bought my first pair of boots from a man who started selling them because his own back felt so much better when he wore them. His spinal fusion surgery had not given him nearly the amount of relief he obtained from changing his footwear.

The same idea of balancing the curves in your back is the reason people use footstools or prefer to stand with one foot up on a step or curb. A brass rail at the bar in taverns and saloons allowed clients to stand more comfortably and, hopefully, stay long enough to order another round.

On one occasion as a young surgeon, I was disconcerted when a hospital patient I was seeing for the first time started to chuckle as I arrived at the bedside. She apologized and told me that she had known who I was before I had introduced myself. My resident had told her that I would be the doctor who immediately put his foot up on the bedrail. My habit of always standing with one foot on a step to relieve my sore back was something I no longer noticed but it was obvious to my sharp-eyed trainee.

**But what do I do when there is nowhere I can stand comfortably?**
You suffer. Suffer with the knowledge that you are doing yourself no harm. I find museums and art galleries difficult. I am often the first one to sit down at a cocktail reception, just to change my posture for a few minutes. I have also caught myself with my foot up on the host's furniture.

Some patterns of back and neck pain are relieved by bending forward slightly. Thus some people find walking in a shopping mall very uncomfortable but they can shop in the supermarket with ease. The difference is the grocery cart. Pushing the cart requires them to bend forward and even provides an opportunity to unload some of their upper weight through their arms. These people can also gain temporary relief by bending forward and putting their hands on their knees, an activity that would make my sore back plead for mercy.

By now I am sure you are getting the message that different patterns of pain require different strategies. Nothing works for everyone, but everyone should find something that works.

# CHAPTER THREE

## *Can You See a Pattern?*

Patients with acute back or neck pain generally come to see the doctor for two overriding reasons. First, they want their pain to stop. Second, they want reassurance that their problem is not dangerous or mysterious. Sadly, the physician's response to the first demand is often to order a series of fruitless investigations that can, in some cases, prolong or intensify the pain. The doctor's typical reaction to the request for reassurance is to provide a long list of the causes of back pain, ranging from the rare and obscure to the spectre of spinal cancer. Unfortunately, this conventional medical approach neither eliminates the acute pain nor reassures the anxious patient.

In the primary care of neck and back pain, the medical model fits poorly. Although many doctors find it difficult to accept, establishing a conventional diagnosis at this early stage is not only impractical, it is unnecessary. It can usefully be replaced by a rapid, symptom-directed approach. I am not describing the assessment of a surgical candidate or the treatment of a chronic, deteriorating spinal condition. Common mechanical neck and back pain are so widespread that they are better considered a human condition than a medical challenge. The increasing popularity of alternative medicine is ample testimony to the inadequacy of conventional medicine's rigid pathology-based approach. Using a simple clinical class-ification is a reasonable first step in addressing the problem.

An effective treatment response should fulfil the patient's needs: pain control and reassurance. The ultimate goal may be the return of function, but the short-term objective is simply the elimination of the pain. For mechanical neck and back pain, this relief can usually be measured in hours to days, not weeks to months. The myth that neck and back pain is inevitably prolonged and disabling is wrong. Most acute episodes subside rapidly. Although there is a high recurrence rate, individual episodes can and should be treated independently. For an overwhelming majority, neck and back pain is benign and self-limiting, and it is best treated without the delay of establishing a medical diagnosis.

A better approach uses a carefully structured history and a confirma-tory physical examination to identify the clinically relevant pattern of pain. Medicine has always used syndromes, a collection of signs and symptoms, to describe conditions for which there is no accepted cause. Approaching neck and back pain as a series of syndromes forms a natural basis for immediate treatment. If the patient's treatment is successful, as antici-pated, this confirms the strength of the original hypothesis.

The four patterns of pain that I will discuss have evolved over the past thirty years. It is not necessary to know the precise physical source of the symptoms to recognize a particular pain pattern or choose the initial treat-ment. In fact, separating these syndromes from their presumed pathology increases their effectiveness.

I take a very pragmatic approach to the early management of mechani-cal neck and back pain. My goal is to provide prompt relief and facilitate the speedy resumption of normal activity. My intention is to treat the symptoms, not the theory. I believe that Pattern 1 is caused by problems within the disc, but my treatment is dictated by specific elements in the history and examination. It has no direct link to the presumed pathology. If Pattern 1 pain were suddenly proven to arise from something other than the discs, that knowledge would not change the clinical presentation of the pattern, nor would it in any way alter the treatment I recommend.

## What exactly does "mechanical pain" mean?

The term mechanical pain indicates pain arising directly from the structures of the spine. It does not include pain that might arise from infection, chemical irritation, or malignant disease. Mechanical pain is a purely physical problem. If your car won't run for a mechanical reason, there is something wrong with the rods and pistons or other moving machine parts. Being out of gas or suffering a computer malfunction would not be considered mechanical causes for the problem.

I teach medical students that mechanical back and neck pain comes from a sore "thing" in the spine. I know they regard this approach as slightly strange, because it doesn't identify specific pathology or relate the pain to a certain illness. My methods don't fit the typical medical model. But they make the point that knowing exactly what the "thing" is does not change the treatment. It is enough to know that the pain arises from some part of the spinal structure. In most cases, knowing how to stop the pain is more important than identifying exactly what part causes it.

## How do you identify mechanical pain?

Mechanical pain responds to movement and position. Move the "thing" and it hurts more. Rest it and it feels better. Load the "thing" and the pain increases. Unload it and the pain subsides. Mechanical spine pain is affected by how you move and how you position your spine. If the "thing" is not severely irritated, merely resting in an unloaded position can eliminate the pain completely. For that reason, most mechanical neck and back pain is intermittent. In more acute situations, resting in an unloaded position will help, but some pain will remain.

## If, as you say, mechanical neck and back pain can be divided into four different patterns, how do you tell one from the other?

The first and most important step is to determine the location of the dominant pain. Without this information, further identification is impossible. Most patients complain of neck and arm or back and leg pain. But the symptoms are rarely of equal intensity. You must identify the single site of the most intense or disabling pain.

My conversation often goes like this:

"Where do you feel your worst pain?"

"In my neck and arm/back and leg."

"If you could choose only one site, where is your pain the worst?"

"In my neck and arm/back and leg."

"You can't have both. You can only pick one: the worst one, the one that stops you from doing what you want to do. Which one do you choose?"

I know that patients find this choice difficult. They think I am missing the point. They have pain in both places. But to establish a pattern, I need to be completely clear as to which of the areas is the site of the dominant pain. Allowing the patient to be vague at this stage will compromise everything that follows.

I consider pain at the top of the shoulder to be neck pain and pain in the buttock to be back pain. Arm-dominant pain exists below the deltoid, the large muscle that surrounds the outer part of your shoulder. Leg-dominant pain exists below the line that separates the bottom of your buttock from the top of your thigh. In the rare case where ambiguity remains, arm or leg pain takes precedence over pain in the neck or back.

### Once you can locate the site of my worst pain, can you tell which pattern I have?

Not yet. There are a few more questions I need to have answered. The second one is almost as important as the first: Is your pain constant or intermittent? There is perhaps no other question in the history for which it is harder to obtain a clear and unbiased answer. Many patients are reluctant to admit that their symptoms are intermittent because they view that as an admission that their problem is not serious. For patients who have been in pain for some time, the individual episodes tend to blur into a memory of an unbroken continuation of pain. But distinguishing between constant and intermittent pain is essential.

When I ask this question, I try to make it very clear that both answers are important and that telling me your pain is intermittent does not diminish my interest or concern. I always explain carefully that I am looking for even short periods when the pain stops, even if returns rapidly. Some patients mistake constant for frequent. What I am trying to establish is if there are any times when the pain disappears long enough for you to be aware that it is gone. The length of time doesn't matter and, as I have said, I know that the pain returns.

Some people tell me that the pain is only gone when they sleep. That doesn't count as intermittent. Other patients tell me their pain disappears only when they take pain medication. This makes my assessment more difficult, but in most cases, unless the patient is taking high doses of a powerful narcotic, I consider the complete disappearance of the pain while taking analgesics to reflect intermittent pain.

This history of continuous pain is so important that I take it in two parts. The first part is: "Although I know it comes right back, is there ever a time in your day when the pain disappears?" If the answer is yes, then I ask the second part of the question: "When you say that your pain stops, does it stop completely? Is the pain totally gone? Does it go to zero?" Often patients will answer yes to the first question and then tell me that although the pain gets much better sometimes, it never disappears completely. I consider that constant pain. The distinction between intermittent and constant pain is critical. Back- or neck-dominant pain that is truly intermittent indicates a benign mechanical problem for which there should be a straightforward mechanical solution.

### How can you be so sure about something as vague and mysterious as neck and back pain?

Mechanical spine pain is neither vague nor mysterious. On the contrary, it is easily recognized and remarkably predictable. Your pattern of mechanical pain is determined not only by your history and my physical examination, but also by your expected rapid response to a specific treatment routine designed for your pattern.

Pain in the neck or back that is caused by systemic disease or some form of cancer does not follow a mechanical pattern and it is never truly intermittent.

**If my pain is constant, does it mean I have cancer or a serious illness?**

Absolutely not! Pain from a previously unrecognized disease or malignancy occurs in less than one in ten thousand people suffering neck or back pain. The most common cause of constant neck or back pain is constant mechanical pain. That "thing" in your back is so irritated that it never completely stops hurting. Constant mechanical pain is more difficult to treat, takes longer to resolve, and is prone to sudden flare-ups, but it is still a benign structural problem.

The rare patient with underlying systemic disease will have a medical history full of clues to a non-mechanical problem. Symptoms such as weight loss, skin rashes, fever, or joint pain in your fingers, toes, hips, or knees may all suggest a non-mechanical source of your pain. Your past health is important, and so is your age. The probability of serious illness increases as you grow older. The chance of having cancer is very different for a sixty-five-year-old man who's a heavy smoker than for a twenty-two-year-old female triathlete.

People with an illness or malignancy will not respond in the predicted fashion to a short course of mechanical therapy. Using pain-pattern recognition and a brief, confirmatory course of physical therapy actually speeds diagnosis of the rare patient with genuine disease.

**My pain is the worst just to the left of my spine at the top of my buttock. It has been there for nearly a month and I notice there are short times, usually when I am walking, that the pain seems to be completely gone. What pattern am I?**

Before I can answer that, I need one more piece of information. I need to know the effect of certain movements on the character of your pain. Does your typical pain, that pain just above your left buttock, increase as you bend forward to tie your shoe? Is it better or worse when you sit in a soft chair?

**My typical pain definitely increases when I do anything that requires me to bend forward. And it is certainly worse if I have to sit for any length of time. Does that help?**

You sound like you have Pattern 1 low back pain. That is the most common pattern. About 75 per cent of low back symptoms are Pattern 1. And Pattern 1 makes up over 90 per cent of the neck-dominant group. You have lots of company.

## What exactly are the characteristics of Pattern 1 pain?

Pattern 1 is neck- or back-dominant pain. That means the pain is felt most intensely, but not exclusively, in the neck or back. Pattern 1 pain is often associated with pain that radiates into the arm or leg, and that is why determining the site of the dominant pain is so important.

Neck-dominant pain includes pain felt in the back of the neck at the base of the skull (the location most people associate with neck pain), pain felt across the top of the shoulder out as far as the shoulder point, and pain that radiates down between the shoulder blades and is felt most strongly in the upper back. Pattern 1 neck pain can cause headaches that can radiate from the back of the head forward, with the aching most intense in the forehead and behind the eyes. Pattern 1 neck pain can be located along the line of the jaw and even into the front of the chest, where it is sometimes confused with heart trouble.

All of these locations represent areas of what is technically called referred pain: pain that originates in that sore "thing" in your neck but which is felt some distance away. The example of referred pain that most doctors use is the pain of a heart attack: pain that arises in the heart but is felt mainly in the arm. Referred pain is not the same as the pain that travels along a pinched nerve. Pattern 1 pain does not directly involve the nerve.

In the low back, Pattern 1 pain can be felt along the spine anywhere from the ribs downward, in the buttocks as far as the upper thigh and into the mid-line tailbone. Pattern 1 back pain can also be referred to the side of the pelvis on the outer aspect of the hipbone, or radiate into the groin and genital area. Distinguishing back- or neck-dominant pain from leg or arm pain may not be as easy as you suppose.

Pattern 1 is the only pain pattern that may be either constant or intermittent. The consistency of the pain will not change the pattern identification, but it will affect the type of treatment and the duration of the symptoms.

Pattern 1 is made worse by bending forward. In the neck, this means looking down, resting your chin on your chest. In the low back, this includes everything from shovelling, raking, and vacuuming to making the bed, picking up the groceries, or tying your shoes. There are very few things you do during the day that do not require you to bend forward. Because everyone tends to slump when they sit, Pattern 1 patients find sitting difficult, particularly in chairs without adequate low back support. These symptoms are reflected in the typical story I hear from a Pattern 1 low back patient. Most of them would rather walk slowly than stand still and they would rather stand still than sit down.

Pattern 1 can be divided into two groups: fast and slow responders. A Pattern 1 fast responder is a patient whose back pain is increased on bending forward but is substantially decreased by arching backward. In the neck, this pain-relieving movement is called retraction, and it means drawing the head backward while keeping the eyes level. It is a movement that requires considerable practice, and one I will discuss in more detail in Chapter 5.

Pattern 1 slow responders feel their pain increase as they bend forward (all Pattern 1 patients do), but their pain also increases as they arch their back or retract their neck. The pain on extension can be more intense than the pain they feel when they bend forward. This is a difficult group to treat, because movement in both directions hurts.

The physical examination should support what I heard in the history. In establishing the correct pattern, the information from the history takes precedence and the examination need only confirm what I already suspect. For Pattern 1, the patient should be able to locate his or her pain with a finger by pointing to one of the areas that represent neck- or back-dominant symptoms. This typical pain will be increased when the spine bends forward. That may require a single movement or several repetitions before the discomfort appears. My purpose in reproducing the typical pain is not to inflict unnecessary discomfort but simply to confirm the presence of Pattern 1. Arching backward or retracting may either increase or decrease the symptoms, and this difference is the basis for separating the fast from the slow responders.

When I test the power, reflexes, and feeling in the arms and legs, I should detect no abnormalities. There should be no loss of function, as Pattern 1 has nothing to do with direct nerve involvement. Unfortunately, the examination may temporarily increase the severity of the pain, and separating pain-inhibited movement from true weakness can be difficult.

A clear history, supported by the findings on the physical examination, will give me all the information I need to recognize Pattern 1 and recommend appropriate mechanical therapy.

### What are the characteristics of Pattern 2?

Pattern 2, like Pattern 1, is back- and neck-dominant. That means the possible pain locations are the same. Pattern 2 is considerably less common than Pattern 1, accounting for about 15 per cent of back-dominant patients, and only 1 or 2 per cent of those with neck-dominant pain.

Pattern 2 is always intermittent. A history of truly constant pain eliminates the possibility of Pattern 2. Pain is intensified by arching backward or with cervical retraction. It is never made worse by bending forward or holding a forward-bent position.

As these patterns were developed, it became obvious that confusion could arise in choosing between a Pattern 1 slow responder and a Pattern 2. Of course, a Pattern 1 slow responder would have pain on both flexion and extension while the Pattern 2 patient would have pain on extension only, but this distinction was frequently overlooked. And if the Pattern 1's extension pain was worse than the flexion pain, then the resemblance to Pattern 2 was even more pronounced. But the difference between the two patient groups is significant and the distinction must be made. Pattern 1 slow responders require a different mechanical approach and are generally more challenging to treat. Managing them as Pattern 2s will eventually make them more painful. The average Pattern 2 patient can easily control the symptoms with a few stretches and minor posture adjustments.

As in Pattern 1, my physical examination of a Pattern 2 patient will detect no problems with the nervous system; no weakness, reflex changes, or sensory loss. The movement testing will elicit the usual symptoms on extension only, and neither repeated forward bending nor holding a flexed position will increase the typical pain.

## You haven't mentioned tests where you bend to the side or rotate. Aren't those movements important?

The movements are certainly important if they produce the typical pain, and modifying them may be part of the treatment. But they do not help differentiate between Pattern 1 and Pattern 2. Both patterns may cause pain with rotation, and both may affect the way you bend to one side. However, the typical trunk shift that is sometimes seen with severe low back pain is almost always associated with Pattern 1.

## What about Pattern 3?

Both Pattern 3 and Pattern 4 are leg- or arm-dominant. That means the pain is most intense below the buttock or radiating down from the upper arm. It does not mean that the pain is in the leg or arm only. Most Pattern 3 sufferers have significant additional pain somewhere along the spine.

Pattern 3 pain is always constant, either at the time the patient seeks medical attention or for a substantial period in the recent past. Both the arm and leg pain must be affected by movement or position of the spine.

Pattern 3 indicates direct nerve-root irritation, and technically, the pain is now called "radicular" rather than "referred." The pain is felt particularly along the course of the irritated nerve and will generally travel to one or two specific areas. Generalized arm or leg pain is more often associated with the referred pain from a back- or neck-dominant Pattern 1 or Pattern 2.

The pain of Pattern 3 is usually very severe although rarely, nerve-root compression can occur painlessly. The typical leg pain, correctly called sciatica and reproduced by the straight leg-raising test I will describe, is intense. Patients with full-blown Pattern 3 pain may have no option but to spend most of their time at rest, unable to participate in their normal activities.

Like Pattern 1, Pattern 3 can be divided into two subgroups, the fast and slow responders, although in this case, fast responder is a relative term. Fast responders can gain some relief in their arm or leg pain with certain

positions of the spine. For the slow responders, no position helps and everything seems to make the pain worse. All Pattern 3s tend to recover more
slowly than do the back- or neck-dominant groups. Fortunately, this
pattern of true nerve-root involvement occurs in less than 10 per cent of the
neck- and back-pain sufferers.

When I suspect a patient of having Pattern 3 in the low back, I frequently ask that patient to try to do a sit-up. That movement aggravates
the inflamed nerve and increases the leg pain to such a degree that completing the action is impossible. If you can manage to do even one sit-up,
no matter how poorly, it is very unlikely that you have a pinched nerve.

With Pattern 3, the results of the neurological examination will be
abnormal. In the low back, the most common finding will be a positive test
for ongoing nerve-root irritation. To perform the test lie on your back with
both legs out straight. Have someone gently lift the painful leg. In Pattern
3, lifting the leg will increase the typical leg pain. Although the degree of
elevation varies enormously, Pattern 3 leg pain is usually intensified before
the leg is lifted more than sixty degrees, which is about two-thirds of the
way to being vertical. Increasing the back pain without aggravating the leg
pain is not a sign of Pattern 3. It merely shows that lifting the leg irritates
that sore "thing" in the back.

Unfortunately, there is no comparable test of nerve irritation to
confirm Pattern 3 arm pain. For that reason, it is even more important
to obtain a clear history of constant, arm-dominant symptoms.

In both the arm and leg, the neurological examination may reveal signs
of muscle weakness or a change in the normal pattern of reflexes. But it is
common to have a pinched nerve with no loss of power (although there
will be a positive test for nerve-root irritation in the leg), so the history
remains more important than the physical examination.

Many people are concerned that they suffer from Pattern 3 because of
the severity of the pain. Yet the amount of pain is not a reliable guide. Most
back and neck sufferers never experience Pattern 3 pain. If you are going to
carry out these tests, do your best to record your findings as if you were
reporting on someone else. The most accurate tests are the measures of
muscle strength. Don't be misled if your pain inhibits or restricts your

movement; that is to be expected, and it does not indicate Pattern 3. What you are trying to assess is the muscles' real ability to deliver normal power.

For the arm tests, ask a helper to provide resistance against your wrist as you try to bend your elbow upward. Is there a difference in the strength on the affected side? If you are working alone, select several objects of increasing weight and see whether you can lift them as you bend your arm. Is there a difference in the amount of weight you can raise?

A second test of arm strength involves holding your fingers straight out with your hand palm-down. Now have a helper try to bend your fingers at the middle joint. Resist as strongly as you can and see whether there is a difference on the affected side. If working alone, hold your hand at your side and press the tops of your straight fingers against a smooth padded surface. See whether you can resist the outward movement of your arm with the strength of your extended digits. Is there any weakness on the affected side?

There are two tests for power in your lower leg as well. Stand erect and raise your heels so you are standing on the balls of your feet. Raise and lower yourself ten times on both feet and then on each foot separately. Is there a difference in the number of times you can repeat the movement? You are checking for genuine muscle weakness, not a reluctance to move because it hurts. Standing on tiptoe often increases low back pain, but that is not a positive test.

Now try to stand on your heels by raising your toes and arches as high off the floor as you can. See if you can walk that way. Can you elevate the front of both feet to the same height? Again, be careful to separate true weakness from restricted movement due to pain.

Reflexes are another measure of nerve function. The best-known reflexes are the ones at your knees, although for Pattern 3 in the low back these are rarely affected. Sit on a table or bench that is high enough to let your feet hang free and wide enough to support the full length of your thighs. Now, using a moderately heavy, blunt object, such as the spine of a large book, tap the front of your leg just below your kneecap. If the reflex is present and normal, your leg will kick upward in a sudden, involuntary motion. If you obtain reflexes for both legs or for neither leg, the test is probably normal. It is significant only when one reflex is normal and the other is gone. Reflexes may be difficult to test on yourself and having a helper is very useful.

The ankle reflex is more commonly affected in Pattern 3, but it is more difficult to test. The reflex is best demonstrated as you kneel on the seat of a chair with both feet hanging off the edge. Using that large book again, have your helper firmly tap the large tendon behind your ankle. A normal reflex causes your foot to jerk downward. As with the knees, the test suggests a problem when only one of the ankle reflexes is absent. If you are going to try this test alone, the reflex can be obtained when you sit in a chair and cross your legs so that your right ankle rests on top of your left knee. You are now in a position to use that book to strike the tendon behind your right ankle. Repeat the test with your left ankle resting on your right knee.

There are two reflexes that can be tested in the arms. One is at the front (the fleshy side) of your elbow, where you can feel a tendon passing from the biceps muscle in your upper arm to the forearm bones below.

With your elbow bent and your palm up, rest the back of your forearm on a table or the arm of a chair. Strike that tendon with the book or another similar object. If the reflex is normal, your elbow will suddenly bend slightly. The loss of the reflex on the affected side only is a positive test.

The second reflex in your arm is produced by striking the tendon of the large upper arm muscle at the back, the triceps, before it crosses behind your elbow. This is a difficult reflex to obtain. It will be visible only if your arm is completely relaxed with the upper arm supported and the forearm hanging free. You can achieve this relaxation by lying face down on a bed with your arm over the side. In this position, however, it is impossible to test the reflex yourself, and you will require help. Unless there is an obvious difference between the two sides, I suggest that you do not read too much into the test.

Checking the sensation in your arms and legs is much easier but less reliable. Using the end of a paper clip or a wisp of cotton batting, you can gauge whether you have the same appreciation of touch on one side compared to the other. You are attempting to measure a true loss of feeling. All the patterns can produce a "pins and needles" sensation, or the impression that the limb is covered with a stocking or glove that changes the quality of the touch. Pattern 3 and, rarely, Pattern 4 are the only patterns where certain parts of your arm or leg are completely insensitive, which means you feel nothing at all in these places. Differentiating between the two sorts of altered sensation can be difficult, and I strongly advise you not to over-interpret the test results. The loss of sensation associated with Pattern 3 will be quite localized. In the arm, it is usually covers the thumb and index finger; in the leg, it extends over the great toe or the outer border of the foot. A more widespread change in sensation is far more likely to be the unimportant, though annoying, abnormal sensation that accompanies the referred pain of Patterns 1 and 2.

Because Pattern 3 occurs so infrequently, I would expect that for most people, the results of all these tests will be normal. You are probably experiencing nothing more than the arm or leg pain associated with a neck- or back-dominant problem. Even if you think a pinched nerve seems to be the trouble, you can take comfort in the fact that over 80 per cent of patients with Pattern 3 recover fully without aggressive medical intervention.

## So what's Pattern 4?

Pattern 4 in the lower spine also produces leg-dominant pain but, unlike Pattern 3, it is always intermittent. It occurs most often in older patients but it too is uncommon. Pattern 4 describes leg pain that is brought on by activity and relieved by rest and a change in position. Achieving pain control is seldom difficult, since the symptoms rapidly disappear once activity ceases, or if the sufferer is able assume a forward-bent posture like sitting. Patients often describe problems with walking. After a short time or over a limited distance, their legs begin to ache and feel heavy or weak. It is important to locate the site of the dominant pain and differentiate between the leg symptoms and pain in the back. The back pain of Pattern 2 can also be aggravated by walking, and the two patterns must be carefully separated. A careful history is essential to identify Pattern 4, because when the patient is at rest the physical examination is frequently normal, and because there is never a positive irritative test (contrary to Pattern 3).

The Pattern 4 sufferer gains rapid relief by flexing the spine or sitting down. Patients are sometimes puzzled that they can walk for only a short distance in a mall but can shop in the supermarket without a problem. They don't realize that using a shopping cart promotes a forward-bent posture. I have had many patients with Pattern 4 tell me that they were able to ride their exercise bicycle or use their treadmill in an inclined position for long periods but could not walk along the street. This illustrates the value of a flexed posture in controlling the symptoms of Pattern 4 pain.

Like the symptoms of Pattern 3, Pattern 4 is caused by direct pressure on the local nerves within the spine. As you will see in Chapter 4, the different sources of that pressure are thought to be the basis for the contrast between the acute, constant pain of Pattern 3 (caused by the chemical irritation of a ruptured disc) and the intermittent, aching pain of Pattern 4 (resulting from encroachment of the surrounding bone).

Pattern 4 in the cervical spine has characteristics not found in lumbar-area Pattern 4. There are significant anatomical differences between the neck and the low back that account for the marked variation in the clinical picture between these two areas. Because the cord ends just below the last rib, it cannot be affected by anything that happens in the lumbar spine. In the neck, pressure is applied directly to the central nervous system rather than to a peripheral nerve. Squeezing the cord results in increased muscle tone rather than a loss of power. Some weakness may occur in the arms and hands, leading to difficulty in handling small objects or writing legibly, but it is a stiff, spastic gait that often draws attention to the problem. The normal tendency for the toes to curl down when the sole of the foot is scratched is replaced by a reaction where the big toe sticks up and the small toes fan apart. Reflexes in both the arms and legs become more pronounced rather than disappear. Pattern 4 in the neck also tends to appear in older patients. Although it may steadily worsen, it frequently stabilizes before the disability becomes intolerable. Cervical Pattern 4 is the only mechanical pattern for which there is no effective physical treatment. If the symptoms reach unacceptable levels, the management options are almost all surgical.

# CHAPTER FOUR

## *As Little Anatomy As Possible*

I t used to be that training as a doctor meant training in anatomy. Fifty years ago, anatomy was the most important course in first-year medicine, one that took up nearly half of the curriculum. Today, it is taught almost on a need-to-know basis. Medicine has shifted from structure to biochemistry, from dissection to genetics. First-year medical students now focus on understanding disease at a more cellular level.

My experience in patient education has paralleled this shift. My early public lectures were filled with details about the structure of the spine. My audiences were subjected to lengthy discussions about the make-up of the disc and the shape of the interlocking spinal joints. I had even collected a box of vertebrae that I would exhibit during the lectures to give my listeners a better appreciation of what the bones of the back actually looked like. I took my plastic spine model everywhere.

I still believe that education is the most important first step in overcoming back and neck pain. But I now realize that the most important part of the learning process is not a detailed outline of anatomy but a basic understanding of the problems that exist and a sure knowledge that they can be both identified and resolved.

I have adapted my approach, particularly in the area of anatomy, to be more along the lines that most of us take with our computer. For the average user, knowing that Ctrl-Alt-Delete will allow you to escape from a frozen screen is much more important than memorizing the layout of your motherboard. Patients with spine pain are no different. Their basic knowledge of anatomy should have a practical application.

It's actually easier to use the patterns of back and neck pain if you know little or nothing about the specific anatomical sources of the pain. It is enough to understand that some physical component, some sore "thing," is causing the problem.

Over the years, my approach to managing neck and back pain has become increasingly practical and progressively less theoretical. If a treatment works and the patient's outcome can be predicted, then it is useful. The reason it works may be important for future research, but it is irrelevant to the sufferer whose pain has just stopped. Attempting an anatomical correlation may even impair successful treatment. If you believe that your neck pain is coming from the small joints at the back of the spine, then theoretically looking up should increase the load on the joints and the intensity of the pain. Naturally, you would accept a treatment approach that avoided arching your neck backward. But what if arching your neck proved to be your most comfortable position? What if arching your neck on a regular basis not only stopped your pain but appeared to prevent its return? What would you do? Would you go with the theory, and avoid doing the one thing that seemed to give you the greatest relief? Of course not. Or, at least, I hope you would not. Theory is useful when it supports practice, but it can occasionally interfere with sensible clinical management.

One good example is the old caution about sleeping on your stomach. In medical school, I was taught that this was a bad position, because lying on your stomach arched your back and increased the load on your spinal joints. Early in my practice, I had many patients tell me that the only relief they got from their back pain was to lie on their stomach. Faithful to the theories I had learned, I discouraged them from lying that way, and cautioned them about the dangers of compressing their spinal joints. I was telling patients who discovered a way of reducing their back pain that it was a bad thing. I am sure that most of them kept right on doing what felt good and sensibly ignored my useless theoretical advice. I have long since come to the realization that, for mechanical neck and back pain, practical success takes precedence over theory.

### I have been told that my back pain comes from a slipped disc. What exactly is that?

Correcting the myth of the slipped disc is one of the best reasons to provide you with a basic outline of spinal anatomy. Discs don't slip. The spine is one of the strongest and most resilient structures in your body. It is able to withstand enormous amounts of force and load. Its structure is designed to provide flexibility and strength in a way that all our technology has not yet been able to duplicate.

### Spine – lateral view

*Each section – cervical, thoracic, and lumbar – is numbered from the top down. T6 is the sixth bone from the top in the pile of twelve thoracic vertebrae. The ribs are not shown but the small ovals that mark their attachments are visible over the entire thoracic area.*

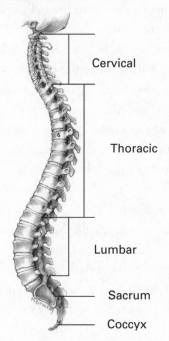

Cervical

Thoracic

Lumbar

Sacrum

Coccyx

The basic building block of the spine is the vertebra. These drum-shaped bones are stacked on top of one another. The first seven below the skull make up the cervical spine. The next twelve running behind the chest form the thoracic spine. The last five in the low back are the lumbar spine. There are, in fact, eight to ten more vertebrae below that. Five of these have fused together to form the solid bone at the back of the pelvis, called the sacrum. The rest hang below the pelvis as the tailbone, or coccyx. Except for the first two cervical vertebrae, all the vertebrae have very much the same shape and, except for the coccyx, they tend to get larger as you move down the spine.

To simplify discussion, the vertebrae are labelled from the top down with a letter and a number. C5, for example, represents the fifth-from-the-top cervical vertebrae. T7 is the seventh bone down in the stack of twelve thoracic vertebrae. Most low back trouble occurs between L4 and S1: in other words between the fourth lumbar vertebra and the first of the five fused sacral bones.

Attached to the back of each vertebra is a bony tube through which the spinal cord and the spinal nerves pass from the brain to the pelvis. Attached to the back of the tube are bony projections that form interlocking joints linking the vertebra above to the vertebra below. They are usually called facet joints. In the neck, the joint surfaces are flat and their movement is like rubbing your palms together. In the low back, the joints take on an L shape. You can get some idea of their movement by bending the fingers of each hand to ninety degrees, then stacking one hand over the other with your fingers pointing in opposite directions. Only a slight rocking motion is possible. The amount of movement in the lumbar joints is restricted, but the stability of the connection is greatly enhanced.

The internal structure of the spinal joints is the same as the internal structure of all the other moving joints in your body. The opposing surfaces are extraordinarily smooth and self-lubricating. In terms of size and function, the spinal joints are very much like the joints at the end of your fingers, and they can crack, just like your knuckles. But, just like your knuckles, cracking your spinal joints never pulls them completely apart or rearranges their positions. Separating the joints slightly releases nitrogen gas dissolved in the joint fluid. It is the same effect as taking the cap off a pop bottle.

**Lumbar vertebra**

*The facets in the lumbar spine are L shaped for added stability. The joint surface of the superior facet faces backward and inward to fit against the surface of the inferior facet above, which points forward and outward. Muscles attach to the transverse and spinous processes.*

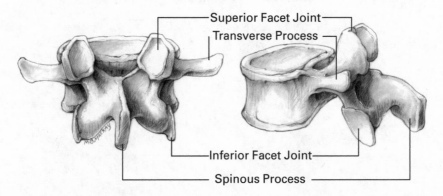

Superior Facet Joint
Transverse Process
Inferior Facet Joint
Spinous Process

## So where do the discs fit, and why don't they slip?

The discs act as shock absorbers between the flat surfaces of the drum-shaped vertebral bodies. The disc itself is made up of an outer layer – containing a dense weave of fibre and cartilage – and an inner centre that, in early life, has the consistency of chewing gum. Although people describe the disc as if it were made of two separate parts, the structure is actually more like a cross-section of a green melon. The centre is softer than the outer shell, but there is no distinct line separating the two. The chemistry of the disc allows it to absorb a large amount of water from the bloodstream. There is no free water inside the disc. It is held in a sugar-protein complex similar to gelatin.

The disc is attached to the vertebrae above and below by an elaborate system of fibres that extends right into the substance of the bone. It is actually easier to break through the bone next to the disc than to tear the disc loose. And even if a small portion of the attachment were to be damaged, the remaining connections would prevent the disc from slipping out of place.

The exceptions to this design are the fused sacral vertebrae, which contain no discs, and the first two cervical vertebrae. C1 has a smaller body (the drum-shaped part) and looks more like a knobby ring. Because it

### The first three cervical vertebrae

*The skull rests on the joints of C1. The tip of the peg projecting upward from C2 is visible at the front of the spinal canal above the posterior arch of C1. The first disc in the spine appears between C2 and C3.*

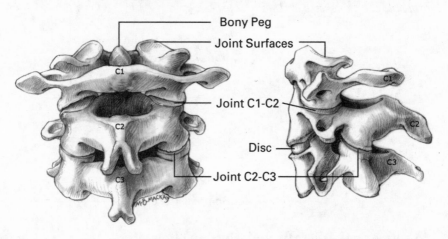

supports the skull, it is named the atlas, after the Titan in Greek mythology who bore the earth on his shoulders. There is no disc between the skull and C1. C2, the axis, has a bony peg at the front that points up like a finger into the ring of C1. This post is bound to the inner surface of the front of the ring by a dense and extremely strong set of ligaments. There are joints between C1 and C2, but no disc. The first disc-joint structure is found between the second and third cervical vertebrae. Because of the unusual structure of C1 and C2, much of your neck movement takes place at these levels. Over half of the movement of nodding "yes" takes place between the skull and C1. Over half of the movement of shaking your head "no" occurs between C1 and C2.

### It sounds like a well-designed system. Why does it hurt so much?

The system is well designed and extremely strong. In addition to the cable system that binds the discs to the vertebrae, the interlocking joints are surrounded by tight capsules firmly attached to the adjoining bony projections. Further strength comes from connecting ligaments and the application of several layers of muscle attached directly to additional bony projections: the transverse and the spinous processes that protrude from each vertebra.

But the spine is subjected to the same stresses and changes of age as the rest of the body. Beginning in your teens, the high water content of the disc begins to diminish, and the formerly superb hydraulic shock absorber begins to fail. Although the fluid within the disc is replenished daily, the balance gradually shifts and the internal environment dries out. As the disc dries, it also narrows, and the narrowing puts extra strain on the outer shell, which may then bulge or crack. The outer portion of the disc is highly sensitive to pain, and stretching or tearing this surface hurts. At the same time as the disc is showing the effects of age, the small joints are beginning to roughen and wear. Just as hips and knees may cause trouble later in life, so too may the small spinal joints.

The whole process is exaggerated by a loss of muscular support along the spine due to lack of exercise and a sedentary lifestyle. Weakness can also occur when the muscles remain inactive because of chronic neck or back pain. Refusing to use your sore neck or your sore back can, in fact, make matters worse.

Weak muscles hurt, but they are not the primary source of back pain. The trouble is with the mechanics of the discs or joints. The sore muscles are just part of your body's response. The only time the muscles cause pain on their own is when they are injured directly, for example, when you get hit on the back.

**It sounds like I am headed for the scrap heap. Is there any hope?**
You are not an old piece of farm equipment rusting in the field. Your body is capable of remarkable repairs. Although the disc dries and narrows (one of the major reasons that we grow shorter as we grow older), it also stabilizes. The effect is to prevent further painful bulging of the outer shell. The cracks and fissures slowly heal and, over time, the drier, thinner disc becomes pain-free.

The small joints also become stiffer and less prone to pain. The rough joint surfaces smooth themselves out, and although they are not as slippery as they once were, they can permit pain-free movement.

The vertebrae themselves will change shape, growing bony projections usually called bone spurs that aid in the process of stabilizing the spine, and increase the amount of contact surface between the bones. More surface means less pressure on any single point and, again, less pain.

### I have heard of bone spurs. Are you telling me they don't cause trouble?

Bone spurs are technically called osteophytes and they are not unique to the spine. They are easiest to observe around the finger joints in older people. Those cartoon witches with knobby fingers are exaggerations of a real condition. Bone spurs can form near any moving joint. Along the spine, unless their size is causing a local problem, they do not need to be removed. Although they can appear impressive on X-rays, and occasionally cause problems by taking up space within the spinal canal, once they are formed, they do not hurt.

### If I wait long enough, will the spine repair itself?

In most cases it will, but as good as the repair process is, things can go wrong. The dry discs don't always stabilize in the best position, and sometimes an older spine can develop a side-to-side curve called scoliosis. The small joints may not stiffen as they should and, in a few cases, they can become looser as they wear. Instead of having less pain, you may experience more.

The highest incidence of back and neck pain occurs in the early forties. There is a second period of trouble, particularly for women, in the early sixties. And, of course, it's possible to have a problem with a worn joint or a bulging disc at any time from your teens onward. Fortunately, the natural history of back and neck pain is to diminish as we grow older. Although you can expect recurrences throughout your life, the ultimate result is generally less pain. There is nothing you can do to prevent advancing maturity, but you can do a lot to minimize its effects. Ageing doesn't have to impair your function, limit your activity, or destroy your life.

### But what about a pinched nerve? How does that get better?

Pinched nerves are quite uncommon. The nerves may be squeezed by a slow bony growth that takes up space within the spinal canal, or by the sudden bulging of a disc. As the nerves exit the spine, they cross directly over the back edge of the disc. A bulge at that point can compress the nerve.

Disc bulges are different from bone spurs, because the disc bulge is accompanied by a strong inflammatory reaction. Inflammation is that redness, tenderness, and heat that surrounds a cut on your skin. A bulge or tear of the disc creates inflammation through rapid chemical reactions. It is the combination of this inflammation and the local pressure that causes the pain.

Nerve roots separate from the spinal cord and leave the spinal canal through exit holes called foramina, between the vertebrae, one on each side, at every level. In the neck and thoracic spine, the nerve roots leave the canal in an almost straight line. The spinal cord normally ends in the upper lumbar spine, just below your ribs. Beginning several levels above that point, the nerves that leave the cord do not exit the spine immediately, but travel downward in the spinal canal as a mass of fibres that the early anatomists called the "horse's tail," or cauda equina. The nerves leave on a gentle slope, and the point at which they may be pinched can be some distance away from where they exit the canal. Because the spinal cord takes up most of the available canal space in the neck and thoracic spine, bulging discs or bone spurs in both these areas may cause quite different problems than they produce in the low back. Pattern 4 in the neck is very unlike Pattern 4 in the low back.

## So where do the different patterns of pain come from?

The relationship of back pain to specific anatomy, ageing, or presumed pathology is only theoretical. We have come a long way in the past twenty years in understanding why back pain occurs, but there are still many things that we do not know. Despite our technology, we can identify a specific source of back pain responsible for a particular attack in less than half the cases. Some things, like a pinched nerve, are relatively easy to diagnose. Others, like neck-dominant pain, still leave us guessing. It is because there is a gap between what science suspects and what practical experience shows that I believe the patterns are so valuable.

**I understand that. But I still want to know what causes Pattern 1.**
Pattern 1 is probably the result of pain arising in the outer shell of the disc.
Pain is produced when the disc is loaded: when you bend forward, lift, or
sit, for example. The shell of the disc is supplied by a branch of the nerve
that exits the spine at that level. Pain from the disc shell is felt not only in
the back or neck, where it is most pronounced, but also in the shoulder,
buttock, or any of the other areas affected by the referred pain of Pattern 1.

Although the theory regarding the origins of Pattern 1 is strong, it is not
guaranteed and it is frequently impossible to identify precisely which disc
is causing the trouble in a particular case.

### Pattern 1

*The* probable *source of Pattern 1 pain is a rapid or extreme distortion of the
pain-sensitive outer disc shell. The pain arises from the disc itself with no
significant intrusion of material into the spinal canal or involvement of a
nerve root.*

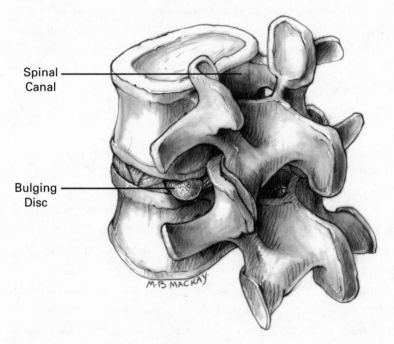

Spinal Canal

Bulging Disc

M·B·MACKAY

## What about Pattern 2?

Pattern 2 seems to arise from the small joints, their capsules and linings, and the associated ligaments. The joints, like the disc, are supplied by a branch of an exiting nerve. Once again, the pain is felt mainly in the back or the neck, but may also be referred to the buttocks, groin, shoulders, and head, for example. Because the pain is produced on extension, and this is the movement that increases the load on the joints, the theory seems reasonable. But some researchers believe the small joints never cause any pain at all. No matter who is right, there is no doubt that Pattern 2 exists.

### Pattern 2

*A* possible *source of Pattern 2 pain is wear in the posterior facet system. These joints have the same composition as the hips or knees and are therefore subject to the same process of osteoarthritis (joint deterioration related to advanced maturity). If it can hurt in the hip, why not in the back?*

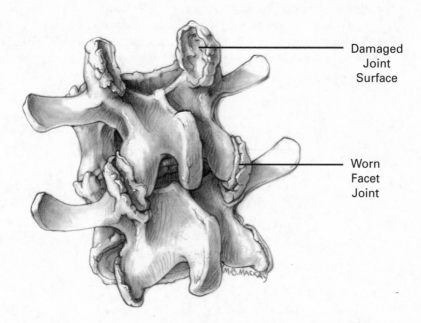

Damaged
Joint
Surface

Worn
Facet
Joint

## And Pattern 3?

When a nerve is directly involved, the diagnosis is easier. There is little disagreement between the pattern and the theory. Pattern 3 describes the result of inflammation and direct nerve compression following a disc rupture. The resulting leg-dominant pain, called sciatica, can be extremely severe. Because the disc has bulged and/or ruptured, Pattern 1 (disc pain) often accompanies Pattern 3 pain, although the leg pain will dominate when the nerve is acutely inflamed.

Anatomical knowledge does provide an answer to a couple of questions. Why can some people have a pinched nerve without severe leg pain? The answer seems to be that the pressure on the nerve is applied to an insensitive portion, and is sudden and sufficient enough that the nerve loses its ability to transmit pain signals. The nerve is numbed, and the

### Pattern 3

*The almost certain source of Pattern 3 pain is direct pressure from a ruptured disc on a nerve root. Decreased water content in the disc creates fissures that weaken the structure and disrupt the outer surface. Notice that one disc fragment has broken loose and is lying free in the spinal canal.*

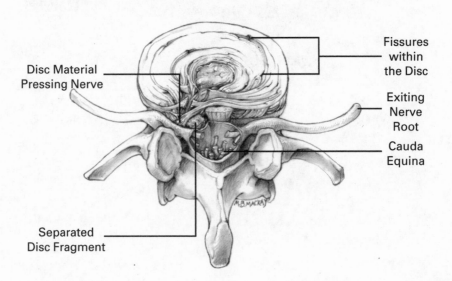

Fissures within the Disc

Disc Material Pressing Nerve

Exiting Nerve Root

Cauda Equina

Separated Disc Fragment

power, reflexes, and sensation are impaired. Very rarely, these individuals may feel only back pain, because the nerve's signalling capabilities are completely shut down.

Most often, Pattern 3 leg pain is made worse by bending forward. But the leg pain can occasionally be aggravated with extension. Why should that be? If the disc bulge isn't at its typical location at the back edge of the disc, but occurs to the side and fills the hole where the nerve exits, then arching the spine backward, a movement that closes the hole, will trap the nerve between the bone and the bulging disc. Bending forward enlarges the size of the exit hole and reduces the pressure.

One case of using anatomy to understand the pattern is the sequestrated (meaning separated) disc. Occasionally when a disc bulges, part of the bulge will actually break loose and lodge in the spinal canal, usually in the exit hole. Patients who experience sequestration often first notice severe, back-dominant pain, a typical Pattern 1. Suddenly, perhaps within a matter of minutes, the back pain disappears and is replaced by severe leg pain. They have become Pattern 3. But it is an unusual Pattern 3, since the leg pain is aggravated by arching backward, not bending forward. Presumably, Pattern 1 appeared when the disc bulged. It then disappeared when the bulging portion of the disc tore loose and the tension on the disc shell was relieved. Pattern 3 began as the fragment lodged against the exiting nerve root, producing both pressure and chemical irritation. The unusual symptom of increased pain with extension is caused by the location of the separated fragment.

## Does this bring us to Pattern 4?

The technical term for Pattern 4 is neurogenic claudication. Claudication means limp, as in a painful walk, not as in droopy. Neurogenic means the problem is in the nerve. In this case, the problem arises because the nerves are compressed by the bony walls of the spinal canal. There is no associated inflammation, and therefore no sign of the acute nerve-root irritation seen in Pattern 3.

Nerves and muscles require blood to bring them energy. Like muscles, nerves require more energy when they are active. If a nerve is tightly

## Pattern 4

*The usual source of Pattern 4 pain is long-standing compression of the nerves travelling in the spinal canal or exiting between the vertebrae. Pressure is applied by bony bars or spurs that grow along the edge of a dried, shrunken disc, or that enlarge the surfaces of a worn joint.*

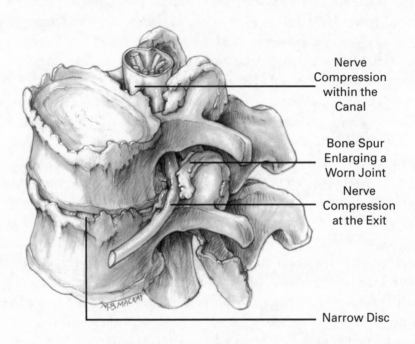

Nerve Compression within the Canal

Bone Spur Enlarging a Worn Joint

Nerve Compression at the Exit

Narrow Disc

compressed within the spinal canal, its blood flow is restricted. The nerve may have sufficient energy to function at rest, but when it is called on to increase output, perhaps to power the legs while you walk, the blood supply is inadequate, and the nerve cannot function correctly. This is the cause of the intermittent leg pain, and often of transient muscle weakness as well.

Doctors use a medical term: spinal stenosis. Stenosis means narrow, and the term relates to the narrowing of the spinal canal. A narrow canal is usually the result of ageing, as bony spurs take up the available space but occasionally, people are born with a small tunnel. Spinal stenosis can certainly be a cause for Pattern 4, but not everyone with spinal stenosis gets into trouble. Sometimes, even though the space is tight, the nerves still function normally. Patients are sometimes frightened unnecessarily by a CT or MRI report that describes "severe spinal stenosis." They may be referred to a surgeon, not because of their symptoms, but because of the imaging study. I don't operate on X-rays. If my patient has no evidence of Pattern 4, neurogenic claudication, then there is no reason to decompress the spine. Regrettably, there are patients who undergo needless surgery to enlarge the spinal canal. Their real problem, often simple mechanical back-dominant pain, remains.

## Can you combine more than one pattern in a single patient?

Yes, you can, but in most cases, one pattern takes precedence. When the choice is between neck- or back-dominant pain, and pain that is most pro-nounced in the arm or leg, it is the arm or leg pain that is considered more important. This pain generally represents direct nerve-root involvement. Occasionally, patients will have more than one problem yet be unaware of the second pattern. I remember operating on a man for acute Pattern 3 leg pain. He had a large bulging disc, and in order to remove it, I had to take off a good portion of the bone on the back of the spinal canal. A couple of months after surgery he told me that not only had his severe leg pain dis-appeared but he was now able to walk as far as he wanted without having to sit down to relieve his leg cramps. This man had been a Pattern 4 patient before I saw him. My surgery to correct the Pattern 3 pain had serendipi-tously solved a problem I didn't even know he had.

# CHAPTER FIVE

## *What Can I Do Right Now?*

The chances are that as you read this book, you are reasonably free from significant neck or back pain. Of course, it is possible that in the midst of your agony, you are clutching this book in desperation. Either way, most people who ask for a consultation come looking for an immediate solution to their problem. So let's get to it.

**Is there something you can do to stop my pain?**
There are a number of things I can do to help you control the pain. In fact, we have already started. The first thing that you need to know is that most neck and back pain disappears quickly and leaves no permanent limitation. Fighting pain is challenging enough, but when you also have to fight unnecessary fear, things get worse. Some of your anxiety will be relieved just knowing that back pain is not a disease and no matter how much it hurts, the pain in your neck or low back is very rarely the mark of a serious problem.

**You say my pain is not serious, but it hurts so much that I've had to stay home from work, and I don't think I can stand it much longer. What do I do now?**

Some very simple things. Although back pain is seldom initiated by the muscles, muscle pain is a significant secondary feature. Patterns 1, 2, and 3 all come with sore muscles.

The first strategy is to move. Stretching the muscles by moving your head or walking around often helps. Staying active rather than staying in bed may seem nonsensical at first, but it works. I am not talking about building a new stone patio or chopping firewood, but about taking a slow walk to the end of the driveway and back, or even around the kitchen table a couple of times. Stay on level ground and walk slowly, but keep moving.

Your body has a complex method of registering pain, and sometimes a strong sensation from one source can block out intense pain from another. This principle of counterirritation has been recognized for hundreds of years, and it still works. Rubs and liniments can help a sore back or neck feel better, at least temporarily.

A heating pad can help, but it may be no more effective than a cold pack or a bag of frozen vegetables. The idea is to find a counterirritant that reduces your pain, presumably by interfering with the pain's access to your brain's reporting centres.

## So is ice or heat better?

Whatever works is best. Neither the heat from the hot pack nor the cold from the ice pack penetrates more than few millimetres into your body. In spite of the claims made in advertisements and all the lovely animations, deep heat actually goes nowhere.

Since different people respond to counterirritation in different ways, there is no hard-and-fast rule. I generally recommend ice in the summer and heat in the winter, because that is what most people like. There is an old joke about a doctor who recommends an ice pack for his patient's bad back. On the way home, the patient stops for some groceries, and while he talks to the girl at the checkout counter, she recommends he try heat instead. He takes the clerk's advice and, much to his relief, the heat works perfectly. A week later, he sheepishly reports what he has done to his doctor, and the doctor is understandably upset.

"You shouldn't have done that!" the doctor snaps. "The waiter at the country club said it had to be an ice pack."

The point is that the result is all that matters. You have nothing to lose by trying both remedies and picking the one that suits you.

### What about a hot bath or a cold shower?

A cold shower could certainly take your mind off your back pain, but too much cold can generate muscle tension and increase your symptoms. I have had many people tell me that their back spasms began when they stood in front of an air-conditioning duct, or when they left the house on a frosty winter day. Although a cold pack may feel good, use it in moderation. The same is true of heat, by the way. Applying heat for too long can damage the skin and cause a fluid build-up in the tissue that can increase the pain. If you are going to use the shower, I suggest you try a warm shower first. Standing may be more comfortable if you can put your foot up on a raised surface. If your shower doesn't have one, try bringing a small wooden stool in with you.

As far as the hot bath is concerned, the warmth of the water may feel good, but your posture in the bathtub will almost certainly be uncomfortable. A bathtub pillow or similar device might help, though sacrificing comfortable posture for a little heat seems a poor exchange. If your pain is lessened when you lie on your stomach, the practical difficulty of achieving the desired posture in the tub may be insurmountable. How will you get out if your back goes into spasm?

A hot tub or a whirlpool bath can provide considerable benefit without requiring you to adopt a posture that would load your back unnecessarily. Stretching out in a hot tub or lying with your back against the jet of a whirlpool is certainly excellent emergency treatment if you have those facilities at hand.

### What about massage?

Massage and manipulation are slightly different. Massage implies a repeated squeezing of the muscles. It can be uncomfortable initially, but it often ends up feeling very good. Massage makes no claim to change the structures of your spine. Although a few massage therapists allege it provides additional health benefits, the primary goal of massage is to alleviate muscle tension and thus reduce your pain. Having a friend or family member rub your neck can be helpful. A professional massage is more involved, but may be worth it.

The outcome should be rapid relief. If a treatment works, that's good. If, after a few sessions, massage has no effect or has made matters worse, that's bad. You have not done your neck or back any harm, but you are wasting your time and maybe your money as well.

## How is manipulation different?

Manipulation, or adjustment, as the chiropractors call it, is intended to address structure and movement within the segments of your spine. Its goal, like that of massage, is to provide prompt pain relief and for acute mechanical neck and low back pain it is successful over half the time.

Except for surgery, manipulation is the most studied form of back- and neck-pain management. Yet we still don't know for sure what it does or why it works. Chiropractors often talk about reducing subluxations, a condition in which the bones of the spine are supposedly partly out of place. But there has never been evidence – either from clinical examination or from a number of imaging studies – that adjustment produces any change in the relationship of one vertebra to another.

Some believe that the pain relief occurs because stiff joints are put through a full range of movement and perhaps areas of tissue tightness or adhesions are loosened or broken down. Again, there is no evidence that the theory is true. No one has ever demonstrated that manipulation changes joint anatomy or range of movement.

Because of this lack of physical evidence, many practitioners believe that adjustment or manipulation produces some type of neuromuscular effect, changing the way muscles interpret the nerve impulses they receive. Supposedly a spasm is released by improving this communication, or resetting the sensor system within the muscle itself. It is an appealing theory, but one without any supporting evidence.

What is undeniable, however, is that manipulation does relieve acute mechanical neck and back pain in some cases for some people. Still, like massage, any useful result should be immediate, or at least rapid. Continuing treatment without a prompt positive effect, or despite increasing pain, makes no sense.

### Is manipulation safe?

In the healthy low back, manipulation is entirely safe. Your spine is far too strong and stable, and the discs and joints too well-attached, to be damaged or disrupted by someone's efforts to manually twist your back. Manipulation can be performed in a variety of ways; quickly or slowly, gently or forcefully, over a wide range or in a limited fashion. None of these techniques can cause harm. The choice usually depends upon the practitioner's training, or perhaps upon what he or she has found helpful in the past.

Neck adjustment is a slightly different issue. There is an extremely small but clearly documented incidence of blood-vessel damage associated with neck adjustments. Vascular injury may lead to a stroke and, in very rare instances, it can be fatal. The blood vessels involved are usually the pair of arteries that run up the back of the neck and enter through the same hole in the base of the skull where the spinal cord exits. The trauma to one of these vessels occurs in an area just below the skull, where it typically follows a winding course. The proper question is not "Does damage occur?" but "How often does it happen?" No one knows for sure. Estimates range anywhere from one event in every twenty thousand adjustments (a number I do not accept) to one incident in every six million manipulations. That is an enormous range, and it reflects our lack of solid knowledge. The majority of people who have explored this issue put the incidence in the order of one vascular problem for every one-to-two-million adjustments.

### I was told that I need regular spinal manipulations to keep my back healthy and prevent future attacks. What do you think?

While there is evidence that manipulation can eliminate neck and back pain, there is no proof that it has any preventative value. You move the bones of your neck and back every day. Having someone else move them for you adds nothing. Having your pain-free healthy low back manipulated may feel good, and it certainly will cause no harm. Manipulating a pain-free neck may make it feel nice, but it also carries the minuscule risk of a serious complication. In both cases, you should remember that you are paying for a treatment only because it feels good and not because it possesses any legitimate therapeutic value.

### Except for the risk of stroke, is there any reason why I should avoid manipulation?

A manipulation or adjustment is not recommended in Pattern 3 leg pain. Forcefully rotating a disc can accentuate the bulge. There have been cases where adjustment in the early stage of disc protrusion has accelerated the process and hastened the onset of nerve pressure.

In both the neck and low back, manipulation should also not be employed if there is a significant abnormality in the vertebrae. Patients with osteoporosis, a thinning of the bones, should probably avoid having their spines manipulated. The presence of any growth or tumour within the vertebra, or a systemic disease like rheumatoid arthritis that affects the spine, is an absolute contraindication.

### What about traction?

Like massage or counterirritation, traction may help. Or it may not. In either case, the theory that pulling the bones of the spine apart will suck the disc back into place, the way you might suction a blob of toothpaste back into the tube, is completely false. Traction may reduce spasm in the muscles along the spine. It can reduce the load applied to the discs and joints and, if that pressure reduction feels good, then traction is useful. However, it has no lasting effect and as soon as the traction is released, everything will revert to its pre-treatment state. But if the time in traction was a time of comfort, there is no reason to refuse it.

The amount of traction necessary to have any effect in the low back is substantial. Computerized machines and traction tables have been developed to try to increase the amount of pull, but even with these devices, the spine is too strong to be pulled apart. Adding a digital readout justifies an extra charge but gives no guarantee of success.

In the neck, the situation is slightly different. The neck is more mobile than the low back, and because traction here can actually separate the bones slightly, the angle of pull is critical. Patients are often given home traction units; a head halter, pulley, and sand bag they hang over a door or a frame. Because pulling in the wrong direction can increase pressure on that sore "thing," many people have had bad experiences with these devices. Although you cannot do yourself harm, you can certainly increase your pain. Again, the decision depends on how good it feels.

Professionally applied cervical traction may employ elaborate equipment or just the practitioner's hands. He or she may be more experienced at getting the correct angle of pull, but the benefits achieved and the lack of lasting improvement are the same as when you do it yourself.

### What about gravity traction or inversion therapy?

Hanging upside-down may be a way to pass the time if you are a bat, but it does nothing special for the human spine. Whether the effect of gravity is applied while you are upright wearing a harness with your legs hanging free, or while hanging upside-down by your ankles or from the seat of an inverted chair, the pull on your spine is no different than that produced by weights or a motor to create routine, horizontal traction on a table.

### What about putting on a cervical collar or a lumbar support belt?

Most people are surprised to discover that collars, belts, and back braces do not prevent spinal movement. If your goal is to hold your neck or back completely still, you will fail. Not that it matters, since absolute immobility may not stop the pain anyway.

A cervical collar can provide short-term comfort primarily through its aura of protection and the physical impediment to moving too far too fast. Some neck braces may help support the weight of the head. But one of the first rules of overcoming neck pain is to keep moving. The cervical collar tends to have just the opposite effect. Moreover, because the collar appears to offer a safe haven, it quickly becomes a psychological as well as a physical restraint. Removing the collar generally means increasing the pain.

Once the collar has been worn for a week or two, removing it can create a feeling of vulnerability. Getting into a collar is easy. Getting out again can be a challenge.

In the low back, a brace or belt also restricts excessive movement, but it provides neither protection nor complete rigidity. From personal experience, I can testify that wearing a tight belt around your waist when your back is sore feels good. I keep one hanging in my closet for those occasions when a little back comfort is welcome. But you cannot depend on a belt or brace to protect your back, and I do not recommend more than an hour or two of occasional use. If your long-term goal is to keep your back moving, then the brace can't help.

### I agree with everything you say, but I hurt so much I want to go and lie down. Is there a right way to do that?

If you are experiencing neck pain, lying down can be useful if you get the proper support. The rolled towel inside the pillowcase may help. Neck pain and its associated headache are extremely sensitive to position, and lying with a pillow that flexes your chin forward too far will quickly increase your pain. In other cases, removing the pillow and using only the towel will lower your head and neck to the point of comfort. Sometimes, the width of a folded towel under the pillow is enough to raise your head and neck into a comfortable position. Finding the correct elevation may mean adjusting the height by no more than a centimetre or two.

I recently treated one of our nurses at the hospital. He was experiencing severe neck pain causing nasty headaches and even pain referred into his chest that he worried might be his heart. I first showed him that all his pains were coming from his neck. I did this by manipulating his neck into a position that immediately increased his headache tremendously. I'm sure he was impressed with my accurate assessment, but he didn't seem too grateful. Next, I had him lie down in the surgeons' lounge, and I adjusted the height of a few towels under his head and upper back until we reached a point where both his headache and his neck pain virtually disappeared. The final position required folded towels under his shoulders and nothing under his head, so that his neck was actually bending backward. It was not a comfortable position, but it was one that treated his pain. Although he now had a position that provided comfort, his work and home schedule were too busy to allow many opportunities to enjoy this relief. As neck pain generally does, his attack did subside eventually. When it did, we both had the satisfaction of knowing that next time he had the ability to relieve his pain more quickly.

If you are going to lie down to alleviate your low back pain, I recommend one of three positions. The right one for you will depend on your pattern of pain.

The first one, I call a Z lie. Lie on your back and draw your hips and knees up toward your chest. Rest the calves of your legs on the seat of a chair or bench. Viewed from the side, you should now resemble the letter Z. To make the position even more comfortable, try a pillow under your head and another under your buttocks. I find that sliding under the chair so that your knees are further over your stomach or chest sometimes works better. The goal of this position is to relieve your back or leg pain, and its success is measured entirely by how good it feels.

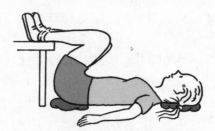

The second position is the exact opposite. Lie on your stomach and rest your upper body on your elbows like a child watching television. If this is too extreme, do the same thing, but place a pillow on the floor under the front of your pelvis to reduce the arch in your low back. If you do not seem to be arching enough, put the pillow under your chest or elbows and increase the amount you raise your upper body.

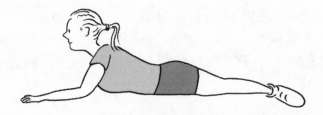

These two positions are completely opposite and yet, for some people, both can provide periods of pain relief. You see my trouble in trying to formulate an anatomical theory that could explain the success of one position without condemning the other. This is one more example of why I favour pragmatism over presumption.

The third position gets you down on your hands and knees. Now you can either arch your back like an angry cat or let it sag like a hammock. Maybe alternating between the two feels good. It's up to you.

**I like your advice so far, but it seems to me that it applies to everyone. Where does treatment based on the patterns of pain come in?**

Right now. We can divide the stages of acute pain management into four steps. The first is education and eliminating unnecessary fear. The second is counterirritation and physical measures to block pain perception and reduce physical strain. The third line of defence is an individualized pain control program based on your particular pattern of pain. I will get to the fourth step, medication, later in the chapter.

Both Patterns 1 and 2 respond to movement, and the key to success is to repeat the pain-control activity frequently throughout the day, preferably every thirty to sixty minutes. The key to managing Pattern 3 is rest. No repeated movement, no matter how appropriate the direction, will soothe an inflamed nerve. The rest, like the activity routines for Patterns 1 and 2, should be scheduled during the day. Only when Pattern 3 reverts to Pattern 1, which it usually will do, does repetitive movement have a place. The emphasis in Pattern 4 is the early introduction of a strengthening program.

I will begin with Pattern 1 in the neck and look at actions you can take when standing, sitting, or lying down. I will also divide Pattern 1 into the fast- and slow-responding groups, since the initial program is different for each.

## NECK
### Pattern 1 – Fast Responder
*Standing*

The pain-control manoeuvre involves an exercise called retraction. While looking forward, draw your head slowly backward so that your ears are directly above your shoulders. At first many people just nod up or down instead of pulling their head back. Imagine your chin as sliding along the top of a table and practise until the movement follows a straight line. You should experience a feeling of tightness at the base of your skull and increased movement in the lowest part of your neck.

Most people find it difficult to learn to retract their neck while they are standing up. They tend to rock through their hips and lower back instead. You should practise standing retractions with your back against a wall to prevent those additional movements. For most people, the exercise is better learned while sitting down.

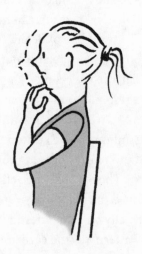

## Sitting

The back of your chair should be level with the lower edge of your shoulder blades. The retraction movement is the same as in standing. You will probably find it easier to perform full retraction by lightly pressing the fingers of one hand on your chin. Their pressure does not replace the action of your neck muscles, but it will help guide the movement, keeping it level and increasing the range.

After you have drawn your head backward as far as it can go, relax and let it slide forward again. The amount of movement is not great, and the action should be performed slowly. You can increase the available movement by letting your shoulders fall backward over the back of the chair. As you retract your head, lower your shoulders and raise your ribcage. If the movement is performed correctly, you will feel your chest rise. Perform five to ten retractions at a session and schedule these sessions as frequently as possible.

## Lying Down

Lie on your back without a pillow so that your head is resting at the same level as your shoulders. In this position, your neck still has its forward curve (lordosis). Look at a fixed point on the ceiling, press your head backward, and draw your chin in. Don't nod; just flatten your neck against the mat. Hold this position for a moment or two and then release, allowing your chin to come forward and your neck to arch. You can check that you are performing this movement correctly by placing one hand behind your neck to feel the squeeze. Gentle traction while lying down relieves tension and may be helpful during an acute episode. It can also be a useful manoeuvre when dealing with cervicogenic headaches, as we will see in Chapter 6.

## Pattern 1 – Slow Responder
### Standing
The ultimate goal in Pattern 1 is to achieve retraction. A slow-responding Pattern 1, however, may find this movement too painful to tolerate, and should therefore begin moving in the opposite direction, an action called protraction. Gently push your head forward, keeping your eyes level and

your chin parallel to the floor. Push to the point of strain, then allow your head to shift back. This movement must be performed gently and only a few repetitions are required. As the range of neck movement improves, the slow responder should attempt retractions. Like all neck-pain control movements, protraction is more easily learned while seated.

### Sitting

Protraction when sitting down is accompanied by a slight forward droop of the shoulders. Keep the head level and avoid nodding. As the range increases or the pain subsides, begin retractions.

### Lying Down

Protraction while lying down consists of no more than thrusting the chin forward. Keep your eyes fixed on a single spot on the ceiling and avoid nodding. Only a few repetitions should be required and, as soon as possible, the Pattern 1 slow responder should begin retractions. Because the pain in this pattern is so easily flared, retractions are best initiated while lying down.

## Pattern 2

### Standing

Pattern 2 neck pain is usually associated with a specific extension movement, such as looking up at the ceiling. Pain control may be as simple as dropping the chin onto the chest. A few repetitions should be sufficient.

Protraction, as described for the Pattern 1 slow responder, may be helpful, and can be combined with a gentle flexion movement. Pattern 2 should be easy to control and should not require many sessions or repetitions.

### Sitting

Both flexion and protraction can be easily accomplished in the sitting position. Flexion can be increased by interlocking your fingers and placing your hands behind your head with your elbows pointing forward. As your chin drops toward your chest, the weight of your arms, with perhaps a gentle downward pull, increases the effect. Relief should come after only a few repetitions.

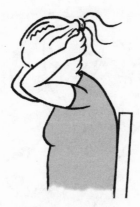

*Lying Down*

Pain control for Pattern 2 seldom requires protraction while lying down. Resting your head on a soft pillow with an adequate cervical support, such as the rolled towel, and then gently dropping your chin forward should be all that is needed.

## Pattern 3

*Standing*

Pain control in Pattern 3 is slower than in the two neck-dominant patterns. The underlying principle is finding the correct position rather than movement. Frequent repetition of any pain-control activity is unlikely to be successful, and can easily increase arm-dominant pain.

Sustained retraction is more effective than repetitive movement. To be more effective the retraction in Pattern 3 is often combined with an additional position, such as a side bend or rotation. Retraction will increase the available range for both rotation and side bending. Retract first then add the additional postures. Experiment with a number of combinations, until you find the one that most efficiently reduces your pain.

*Sitting*

In addition to holding a retracted/rotated/side-bent position, Pattern 3 sometimes responds to brief periods of self-traction. Unfortunately, the pain relief usually lasts only as long as the traction is maintained. Place the palm of one hand under your chin and grip the back of your head with your other

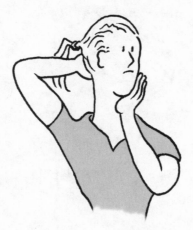

hand. Lift your head up, away from your shoulders. A slight stretch of the neck can produce considerable reduction of arm-dominant pain. Retracting or rotating your head as you apply traction may magnify the benefits.

### Lying Down

The use of a cervical roll is essential. The retraction manoeuvre is the same. The emphasis is on maintaining the best position rather than doing repetitive movements.

## LOW BACK

### Pattern 1 – Fast Responder

#### Standing

Standing up to arch backward is a natural reaction following prolonged sitting. To increase the backward movement, place your hands low on your buttocks and push your hips forward without bending your knees. Keep your head balanced above your shoulders. Try not to move through your hips or just arch your neck. Frequent sessions of five to ten repetitions work best.

#### Sitting

To extend your low back from a sitting position, you must have a seat without a back. Take a firm grip on the sides of the seat to avoid tipping over. Many people find this an awkward exercise, although it has the advantage of eliminating unwanted movement in the hips and knees.

## Lying Down

The passive prone lumbar extension, also called a sloppy push-up, is generally the most effective pain-control manoeuvre for the fast-responding Pattern 1 patient. Begin by lying on your stomach and placing your palms on the floor beside your shoulders. Push up, raising your upper body but keeping your hips against the floor. Your aim is to push up until your arms are straight and you can lock your elbows. Don't let your belt or belly button leave the ground. Keep your chin tucked, and don't use your neck muscles to help raise your shoulders. That can give you a headache. The power comes from your arms, not from the muscles along your spine.

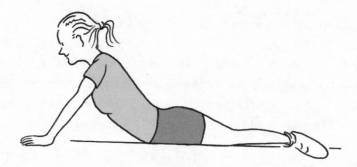

Your range of movement will tend to improve with repetition. It is important to both lock your elbows and keep your pelvis down. Many people find the best starting position is with the hands placed beside the ears, or even above the head, rather than opposite the shoulders. These arm positions require less extension before your elbows are fully straight. As the manoeuvre is repeated and your attainable arch increases, the position of the hands can be slowly brought down to shoulder level.

Concentrate on letting your back sag. Some people find it useful to breathe in at the start of the push-up and exhale once they are in the fully elevated position. Maintain a fixed rhythm. Say to yourself, "Up ... lock ... sag ... down." Having someone apply downward pressure on your buttocks may increase the beneficial effect.

The sloppy push-up generally becomes the mainstay of Pattern 1 pain control. It should be repeated often with five to ten repetitions in each session.

### Pattern 1 – Slow Responder
*Standing*
Gently bend forward with your hands on your knees, taking as much weight through your arms as you can. Keep your knees bent slightly. As you straighten up, bring your body erect before you straighten your legs. Perform the repetitions slowly and avoid sudden movement. Since the goal of Pattern 1 pain control is extension, try arching your back a little as soon as the pain begins to diminish.

*Sitting*
Bend forward and let your chest slump toward your knees. Keep your hands on your thighs and take as much weight through your arms as you can. Straighten by pushing up with your arms rather than by using the muscles in your back. The purpose of this exercise is to increase available range. Since ultimately Pattern 1 patients require extension, this intermediate routine should be used carefully, and only for a limited time.

*Lying Down*
Lie on your back. Draw your knees up over your chest by pulling on the ends of a towel passed behind your knees. The movement is slow and gentle, with your arms supplying most of the power. The purpose of the exercise is to increase low back movement so that you can begin the extension stretches.

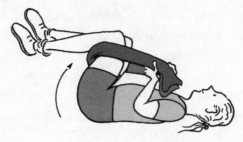

Before Pattern 1 slow responders can perform the sloppy push-up, they must be able to simply lie on their stomachs. Even this amount of extension may prove unacceptably painful. Start by lying over one or two pillows placed under the pelvis. When this amount of extension can be tolerated, decrease the pillow support until you are flat on the floor. Progress to the passive extension exercise gradually and start with the hands placed well above the head.

## Pattern 2
### Standing
Bend at the waist and let your hands drop toward your feet. Don't hurry and don't strain. The goal is not to touch your toes but to reduce your Pattern 2 pain.

Because Pattern 2 is easily controlled, few sessions and repetitions should be necessary.

### Sitting
As you bend forward, put your hands on your knees and lower your chest toward your thighs. To increase the effect, let your hands slide down your lower legs toward your ankles and allow your chest to rest on your thighs, or even slide between them. When you push yourself up, use your arms and avoid tightening the muscles in the small of your back. Imagine your spine slowly uncurling from its C shape, beginning with the lowest section and moving upward.

To add a greater stretch, sit with your legs straight out in front of you before slump forward.

### Lying Down
The simple knees-to-chest exercise described for the Pattern 1 slow responder works extremely well for Pattern 2. Pull your knees tightly to your chest and hold that position for a few moments before letting go. Lift both knees up at the same time. Pulling up one leg alone is less effective, since the opposite leg stabilizes the pelvis and limits low back movement.

Because Pattern 2 is easily controlled, few sessions or repetitions should be required.

## Pattern 3
### Standing
There is no useful pain-control manoeuvre for acute sciatica in the standing position. Most Pattern 3 sufferers find themselves unable to change their standing posture due to the pain. The emphasis in Pattern 3 is on rest in the proper position. Any standing posture that minimizes the leg-dominant pain is helpful.

### Sitting
As a rule, maintaining an increased lumbar lordosis is helpful. Most patients with Pattern 3 leg pain find it more comfortable to sit twisted to one side with the affected leg as straight as possible. Because sitting increases disc load, and because Pattern 3 may be due to disc pressure on the involved nerve, sitting for any period of time generally increases the leg pain and should be avoided, if possible.

### Lying Down
The Z lie position and the prone lying position (the TV position) described on page 74 are both helpful for Pattern 3. The fortunate patients (if anyone with acute sciatica can be called fortunate) gain some relief in both positions. Varying the two positions alleviates the monotony and extends the period during which the patient experiences some leg-pain relief. Although prolonged bedrest is not advisable, frequent rest periods are almost essential. As a general guideline, the Pattern 3 sufferer should spend fifteen to twenty minutes out of each hour resting in the position that provides the most leg pain relief. The remaining forty minutes of the hour can be used to carry out necessary personal functions, household responsibilities, or, for the truly obsessive, the demands of work.

The principle of treatment for Pattern 3 is rest. Although patients are frequently advised to begin an exercise program, this is not appropriate for someone in the throes of acute Pattern 3 sciatica.

## Pattern 4

### Standing

Pain control in Pattern 4 is never difficult. Since the pain is always intermittent and related to using the legs, pain control can be achieved by
merely ceasing the activity. For most Pattern 4 patients, pain relief requires
that they bend forward, resting their hands on their knees, or squatting
down, if they are able. No particular exercise is required.

### Sitting

Sitting and slumping forward brings relief to most Pattern 4 leg pain
within a few minutes. The stretching exercises used in Pattern 2 may be
helpful but are usually unnecessary.

### Lying Down

The key to long-term pain control in Pattern 4 is developing the ability to
perform a standing pelvic tilt. That requires abdominal muscle control
and technique. The tilt is best learned lying down. Lie on your back with
your knees bent and your feet flat on the floor. Flatten the small of your
back against the floor by tensing your abdomen, tightening your buttocks,
and rotating the front of your pelvis toward your chest. Your feet and your
hips should stay down. You should feel the effort in your low back and in
your stomach.

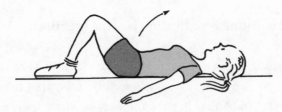

Maintaining the pelvic tilt when you are standing up requires abdominal strength, so the early treatment program for Pattern 4 has a routine of
strengthening exercises rather than pain-control manoeuvres.

### How can I be sure my specific pain-control program is working properly?

Obviously, it is working if your pain is immediately reduced or abolished. But that doesn't always happen. To evaluate the effects of a specific mechanical-pain-control activity, you need to be familiar with the concept of centralization. This phenomenon describes the tendency of back and neck pain to retreat toward the mid-line as it improves. A shift in location toward the centre is a good sign. A shift away from the mid-line into the shoulder and arm or buttock and leg is an indication that the therapeutic activity is not succeeding, and may be making matters worse.

Centralization has become so popular that I have heard some therapists tell their patients that only centralization represents success. The therapists seem disappointed if the centralization process does not occur and the pain simply disappears. I doubt their patients share that regret. The ultimate goal of any treatment is the removal of pain, and centralization is merely a signpost along the correct path.

One element of centralization must be emphasized. After shifting to the mid-line, the pain sometimes intensifies. In this one situation, you really do have to feel worse to get better. The good news is that the increased centralized pain never lasts long. Since it is a new pain in a new location, most patients find it easier to tolerate. A change is almost as good as a rest.

### Earlier, you mentioned medication was the fourth step. When does that come in?

I rarely prescribe drugs on the initial visit for treatment of mechanical spinal pain. Most people do extremely well by following the first three steps. But when pain control is not complete, or where there is a specific need, I will add some form of pain medication.

### Is there a drug of choice?

The Agency for Health Care Policy and Research guidelines recommend non-narcotic, over-the-counter pain relievers. I think this is a very good suggestion. Most mechanical neck and back pain can be rapidly controlled by mechanical means. Resorting to narcotics is seldom necessary. Although the danger of addiction to prescribed narcotics has been overstated, they are still powerful drugs, and may impede normal daily function. Some patients are also very attracted to their soothing effects or by the temporary euphoria they can produce.

### So you never prescribe narcotics for patients with back pain?

Yes, I do, but only in quite special and limited circumstances. My decision is based on a number of factors, but the most important is the necessity of maintaining function. No medication is helpful if all it does is dull a patient's sensibilities without improving activity. Using a narcotic occasionally to stay at work is very different than downing narcotics to stay at home.

### What about anti-inflammatories?

Non-steroidal anti-inflammatory drugs (NSAIDs) have been widely used in treating mechanical back pain. They are usually less effective than simple non-narcotic analgesics, probably because most back and neck pain does not contain a significant element of inflammation. The NSAIDs do have a direct pain-relieving effect, but I generally prefer a simple over-the-counter analgesic. Anti-inflammatories have significant side effects, and there are many cases every year of people who develop serious complications, often gastrointestinal bleeding, because of prolonged use. I would hate to see someone develop a life-threatening condition from medication for a benign, self-limiting, mechanical problem.

### What's this talk about COX-2 drugs? Are they better?

The COX-2 anti-inflammatories were introduced several years ago to avoid the gastrointestinal problems associated with the older types of NSAIDs. The benefits derived from any non-steroidal anti-inflammatory drug are believed to be due in part to their suppression of a particular substance within the body, COX-2. Their serious side effects are thought to come from an unwanted suppression of a related enzyme, COX-1. By targeting only COX-2, it was hoped that these new drugs would be both effective anti-inflammatories and safer to use.

Whether or not they are better, they are certainly more popular. They have become the most widely prescribed anti-inflammatories in the world. There is some concern that their safety record may not be as good as was originally hoped. And there are recognized adverse reactions with other drugs. It is also becoming clear that in many cases they are no more effective than the older medications.

There is certainly nothing wrong with recommending a COX-2 anti-inflammatory drug over a traditional NSAID, but I believe the benefit is marginal and they are more expensive. In any case, no medication, certainly not an NSAID, should supersede the first three steps in dealing with an acute back- or neck-pain attack.

### What about other drugs like steroids, muscle relaxants, or anti-depressants?

Those are all powerful medications. Steroids serve the same purpose as the NSAIDs, which is to reduce inflammation, but they carry an even greater risk of complications. They can be taken orally or injected by a doctor into your spinal canal to deal with a single site of local inflammation. The injections are usually reserved for cases of acute sciatica in Pattern 3, but in some medical centres spinal steroid injections have become popular for treating Pattern 4. Since Pattern 4 shows little evidence of inflammation, the method of action is unclear, but some doctors are convinced that repeated steroid injections help. It becomes a question of weighing the benefits of the injections against the risks, and considering alternatives such as developing a strong pelvic tilt, or surgery.

Muscle relaxants do not merely relax the muscles along the spine. They relax your entire body. Many produce a degree of relaxation that makes intricate work impossible. I certainly would not recommend using a muscle relaxant for your back pain just before you take out your eighteen-wheeler for a trip across the country. Like NSAIDs, some muscle relaxants appear to have a direct pain-relieving effect, but in most cases, my choice would still be a simple over-the-counter pain reliever. I wouldn't raise an objection, though, if someone tells me that they have had great relief with a particular medication, and they are using it correctly.

Chronic neck and back pain has been associated with depression. The idea behind using an anti-depressant is that if you feel better about yourself, you will cope better with your pain. Low-dose anti-depressants can be used to improve sleep. The argument for anti-depressants has very strong proponents as well as opponents. But an anti-depressant for acute short-term neck or back pain is inappropriate, in my opinion. The drugs have too many side effects, and there is no reason for their use in a straightforward mechanical problem.

### Should I try glucosamine or chondroitin?

If you want to. They seem to be safe, but there is no good evidence that they have any useful effect. Glucosamine sulphate (the form in which it is usually sold) and chondroitin sulphate have been advocated for the treatment of osteoarthritis, which is the wearing-out of the joints that inevitably accompanies advancing maturity. They are naturally occurring substances found within the connective tissues of the body and in the cartilage that surfaces the joints. Both are believed to play a role in the growth and preservation of cartilage, but there is no conclusive evidence that either compound prevents or reverses the process of joint degeneration that leads to osteoarthritis.

Their value in treating back pain is even more uncertain. So far there has been only one study that examines the results of treatment for degenerative back problems, and the results neither support nor reject their use. Since their presumed action is on articular cartilage, and since most back pain probably arises from problems within the disc, the study's failure to endorse these supplements is not surprising.

Glucosamine and chondroitin sulphate are not drugs and are not regulated in any way. They are considered nutritional supplements. In one recent independent analysis of commercially available products, nearly one-third failed to contain the stated amounts of the two substances. The shortage was generally in chondroitin sulphate. One possible explanation is that chondroitin (much of which comes from shark cartilage) costs four times as much to manufacture as glucosamine.

Many practitioners recommend combining not only glucosamine and chondroitin but also a variety of other additives such as fish oils, yucca, manganese, and vitamins A, C, and E. I heard one commercial that promoted using glucosamine in a liniment and rubbing it right on your back. It promised pain relief in fifteen minutes as the ingredients went to work repairing your spine. Whether glucosamine works or not, this claim is ridiculous.

Given all the different unproven approaches, questionable quality control, lack of science, and significant cost, I don't recommend these compounds for back pain and continue to favour more straightforward mechanical treatment.

### Your ideas seem very simple. Can it really be so easy?

Control can be simple, but it is seldom easy. Gaining the confidence you need to work through the pain takes a good deal of knowledge and more than a bit of faith. Separating useful physical treatments from those that waste your time and money requires a sophisticated consumer. Selecting the proper pain-control program means correctly identifying your pattern of pain and being willing to invest time and effort to get ahead of the pain.

Patterns 1 and 2 require you to perform repetitive stretching exercises frequently throughout your day. Pattern 3 demands that you rest often and interrupt any normal routine you may have left. There is another problem with Pattern 3: a prolonged period of increased vulnerability. For about two years after an attack of sciatica that recovers without surgery, you retain an increased risk of another episode. The probability of suffering another pinched nerve gradually falls back into line with everyone else's, but for a number of months, you will have to be careful, practise proper back care, and avoid activities that put excessive loads on your spine.

Controlling Pattern 4 means embarking on a long-term program of trunk-strengthening exercises, real exercises that leave you sweaty and short of breath. Many people find it easier just to take a pill or call the chiropractor.

# CHAPTER SIX

## *This Whole Thing Gives Me a Headache*

O
ne of the first things you discover when you start treating neck pain with movement and posture is that if the treatment gives your patients a headache, they are likely to be unhappy with your efforts. Patients are not willing to trade a pain in the neck for a pain in the head. But the two are closely related, and it is remarkably easy for the pain in your cervical spine to spread upward and produce a crashing headache.

The technical term for this, a headache caused by a problem in the neck, is "cervicogenic headache." The exact source of the pain is unclear. One possible cause is a spread of the painful spasm from the muscles in the back of the neck to the muscles that cover the skull. Many people, excluding those who can wiggle their ears, don't realize that your head is covered in muscle, and that the muscle sheet extends from the base of the skull at the back to the muscles that raise your eyebrows. Tension beginning in the neck can spread quickly to involve the entire area.

Cervicogenic headaches could also be considered a form of referred pain. Neck-dominant symptoms can occur along the top of the shoulders or between the shoulder blades. Having the pain in your head may be the same process, but it can be more disabling.

Areas of referred pain can develop local tenderness. The muscles not only transmit the pain message, they react to it. It is common for people experiencing neck pain to feel painful lumps in the muscles across the tops of their shoulders. My personal experience is a tender, walnut-sized lump that appears along the inner edge of my right shoulder blade. Pressing on the lump hurts a lot. If I can get someone to massage it for a little while, the muscle relaxes and the local pain subsides. Of course, since the problem is actually in my neck, the relief is temporary. As soon as I begin to move, the pain and the lump return.

Exactly the same situation exists in the head. Neck-related headaches produce muscle pain and tenderness across the back of the neck and the skull, in the large muscles above your ears and across your forehead. Having your head massaged will identify the painful muscles and probably help temporarily. But, as with my painful walnut, the benefit is short-lived, and as long as the underlying neck problem remains, the headache will return.

Another possible source of cervicogenic headaches is irritation of the nerves that begin in the neck but supply sensation and pain to the back of the head and the face. Injecting these nerves with local anaesthetic has been shown to sometimes stop, or at least greatly reduce, the headache.

Because so many headaches seem alike, defining a particular type of headache and relating it to a specific source is difficult. The International Headache Society has proposed classifications for both cervicogenic and migraine headaches. They also recognize other types of headache. The commonest is a tension-type headache for which no definite cause has been identified. Separating migraine, tension-type, and cervicogenic headaches means listening carefully to the relevant points of the patient's history. The approach is not all that different from diagnosing the correct pattern of neck or back pain.

### My headaches are so severe, sometimes they make me throw up. Am I getting migraines?

A migraine headache is a very unique type of pain. Although they are not rare, they are certainly not the most common form of headache. For many people, the term migraine has become synonymous with severe, and they describe any bad headache as a migraine headache. However, the severity of the pain does not give you the correct diagnosis.

Migraines can make you nauseous, but so can other types of severe head pain. Sometimes the nausea has more to do with the drugs you take to stop the pain than it does with the headache itself.

A migraine headache is caused by inflammation around the blood vessels in the brain and by changes in the blood flow. The reason for these changes is still unknown.

## So how can I tell if my headache is a migraine or not?

The best way seems to be a careful review of the elements of your headache history. Migraines, like back and neck pain, fit into definite patterns.

Here are the essential points. For your headache to be considered a migraine, you must suffer from repeated, intermittent attacks. Each attack can last anywhere from several hours up to three days. Your headache should possess at least two of these four characteristics:

- The headache occurs on one side of your head only.
- The headache is moderate to severe. Mild migraines do occur, but they are rare.
- The headache is aggravated by the ordinary activities of your daily life.
- The headache throbs or pulses. The pain is not steady.

In addition to those elements, the headache must also possess one of the following two features:

- The headache produces nausea or vomiting.
- The headache creates an aversion to light or noise.

Finally, for you to be considered a migraine sufferer, you must have no medical history of a condition known to be associated with headache.

**I have heard that people with migraines see funny lights or even smell strange odours before the headache starts. Is that true?**

The flashing lights, blurred vision, funny smells, and all the rest comprise the aura that precedes the headache. They are produced by the same blood-vessel changes within the brain that will produce the pain. Only about one migraine sufferer in eight experiences an aura. In older classifications, the aura was a mark for what was called a "classic migraine." That term is no longer used, since most experts now believe that a migraine with or without an aura is essentially the same problem.

**I guess I don't really have a migraine, but the pain is still awful. And my neck hurts, too.**

Your last comment is important. Neck pain is one of the hallmarks of a cervicogenic headache. In my practice as a spine specialist, neck-related headaches are the most common type of headache I see. They occur in more than a third of the patients who come to me with neck problems. And it is certainly the most aggravating location for neck-dominant pain.

**Are you saying that if I have both neck pain and headache, my headache is caused by my neck?**

It's not quite that simple. Cervicogenic headache exists, but identifying its pattern requires the same approach that we have used for migraine or the patterns of neck pain. Many people suffer a non-specific headache called a tension-type headache. Although the name implies it is related to tension or stress, the actual causes are not understood. It represents a collection of all those headaches we cannot identify once we have dismissed the ones for which we know the cause, or can at least identify the source.

**Then how can I know I have a headache coming from my neck?**

The first point is the one you have already mentioned. The headache starts in your neck. The pain begins at the base of your skull in the region called the occiput. It is associated with tenderness in the muscles at the top of your spine.

## What are the other features?

The headache begins on one side of the occiput. As it intensifies, it can spread forward. Occasionally, it may spread to cover the whole head, but it never just switches sides.

The headaches usually begin as short periods of pain, but over time, the recurrences begin to last longer and longer. In some cases, the pain can become continuous. The headache can be moderate to severe but it is non-throbbing. It does not stab or pulse.

Although anyone can experience a cervicogenic headache, it is slightly more common in women.

## If you examine me, is there any way you can tell if my headache comes from my neck?

A cervicogenic headache is triggered or greatly aggravated by specific neck movements. It can occur after you have held your neck in one position for a long time. During my examination, I will move your neck and apply pressure to your head in different directions. If doing that gives you a headache, it is probably coming from your neck. Generally, I will also find a restriction in the range of your neck movement and local tenderness when I press on the muscles at the top of your neck just below your skull.

## Is there anything else?

Your history may also include other areas of neck-dominant pain, such as pain across the top of the shoulder or down between the shoulder blades. Cervicogenic headaches themselves can cause a number of other troubling symptoms, such as nausea, dizziness, blurred vision, or even difficulty swallowing. Many of these things can occur for other reasons as well, but a headache from a sore neck may be the only thing you need.

To label your headache cervicogenic, you should not have the criteria listed for migraine or other type of headache, and your medical history should not contain any record of illnesses or other conditions that would account for your headache.

**I can see where separating the different headache types might be confusing.**

It can be. Since the amount of pain is not a guide, telling me you have a bad headache doesn't help the diagnosis. It is the same mistake that people make when they assume that a pinched nerve always hurts more than Pattern 1 or Pattern 2. I understand that the severity of the pain is the main reason that most people seek help, and it is certainly something I consider in the treatment, but it is no help in classification.

Tenderness doesn't help much either. Migraine, tension-type, and cervicogenic headaches can all be associated with sore muscles on the back of the neck and around the shoulders. Only the tenderness at the base of the skull may be useful in spotting the neck-related headache.

**Does stress have anything to do with my headache? I often get a headache when I am driving in heavy traffic, usually when I am late for work.**

Stress has a great deal to do with that headache, but so does the position of your neck. A lot has been said about the negative effect of stress on pain. This relationship is actually a loop, because pain can become a major source of stress. There is no doubt that if you have a headache, being under emotional pressure will make the pain worse. Enduring a headache when you can rest comfortably in a quiet, dimly lighted room is much less exhausting than confronting the same headache in the middle of a high-pressure business meeting, or while you are trying to make up time on your drive to work.

But the stress of driving is not the only reason why cervicogenic headaches can occur. Your posture behind the steering wheel pushes your chin forward and raises your shoulders, tightening the muscles along your upper back and in your neck. Keeping those muscles tight will lead to pain. Once you have neck pain, it can spread up to your head, and there is your headache.

**Yes, here I am with a splitting headache. What can I do about it?**

The steps are the same as the ones I discussed in Chapter 5. Start with understanding the problem and realizing that, although the headache can be severe, it is not life-threatening or permanent. Understanding why you hurt can be a powerful tool for turning down the pain.

The second step involves counterirritants: ice packs, heating pads, or liniments. Massaging the tight muscles of your neck and shoulders can help. So can massaging the tight muscles at the top of your skull and in your forehead.

The longest-lasting relief, however, usually comes from dealing directly with the neck itself. Mechanical neck pain produces mechanical headaches, and so the solution lies in changing the physical situation within the spine.

## How do I do that?

You begin by changing your posture. Sitting hunched in the car with your chin stuck forward is what started your headache in the first place. Reversing that posture and releasing the tension in the tight muscles of your upper neck should be the first step toward recovery.

But be careful! Any attempt to rapidly increase your neck movement, or radically change your posture, can profoundly increase your pain. The mechanical treatment of cervicogenic headache is a game of small movements. Take it easy and take it slow. A little goes a long way.

Your goal is to locate the "escape position": a posture that can sometimes almost magically abolish your headache. Lie down on your back with your head on a small pillow. Put a rolled towel inside the bottom edge of the pillowcase to support your neck. How is your headache now? If the pain is worse, you will need to change your position. This will require raising or lowering the height of the pillow. You may want to remove the roll. The idea is to make the changes in very small stages. Adding the thickness of a folded towel can be enough to increase or decrease the pain significantly. Unlike the neck, where retraction is the commonest pain-control movement, many headaches respond more favourably to protraction. So try building up the height of the pillow before you try reducing it. Remember, one small step at a time.

Move slowly and pause for a minute or two between each change. It's easy to slide right past the escape position and never know you found it.

Because finding the escape position can take a good deal of experi-
mentation, having someone assist with the pillows and towels is a
great help.

**Suppose I build the pillows up so that my chin is almost on my
chest and that doesn't help? If I remove towels and pillows until my
head is flat, the pain is still there. What do I do now?**
Not everyone can find an escape position, but I wouldn't give up yet. If you
have put your neck through as much of a forward range as you can, start
to move it backward by putting towels or even a pillow under your shoulders behind your shoulder blades. You can extend your neck as you are
lying on your back. In each position, stop and wait for a few moments to
see what effect it has on the headache. Be patient and pay attention to the
small changes.

**What if I do find the escape position? What next?**
For most people, the initial escape position is very specific. Moving even a
small distance in either direction will cause the pain to return. Once you
have located the position, the next step is to enlarge it. You do this with a
series of nods.

**You mean like nodding "yes"?**
Exactly, but very gently. Use the type of nod that says you are willing to try,
not one that says you're very excited to go. The idea is to gradually stretch
the tight muscles in the upper part of your neck, the location where the cervicogenic headache probably arises. Begin in the escape position and nod
up and down six times. Now gently protract, that is, stick your chin out.
Don't look up or down. This is not the nod. Keep your eyes fixed on a single
point above your face and move your head forward in a straight line.
Holding a slight protraction, nod six times.

Now move into retraction, draw your chin straight backward. Again,
keep your eyes in a straight line and don't try to go very far. When you have
pulled back a little, do six more nods.

Take a short rest in your original escape position and then do it all over again.

### That sounds difficult. Is there anything I can do to make it easier?

It helps to use a fingertip on your chin to guide the protractions and retractions. If possible, have someone assist you, and watch to be sure that your movements are minimal and correct. Ease yourself into the routine by including your favourite counterirritant – heat, cold, or massage.

### How long does it take?

Once you locate your escape position, you should be able to expand it fairly quickly and gain a degree of headache control within thirty minutes. I always hesitate to give patients a definite timeline. What takes half an hour for one patient may be five minutes for another. Pain control can take hours and, for an unfortunate few, may never occur at all. It's counterproductive to set the alarm for thirty minutes and then give up if you are not successful in that time.

### If I do get my headache under control, how can I prevent it from coming back?

Sadly, you can't. Because so much neck and low back pain is spontaneous, no program can prevent the headache they cause from returning. But you should be prepared with the things you can do to limit the recurrences or reduce the intensity when your headache reappears.

While you are standing, keep your head balanced on your shoulders. Since most neck pain is Pattern 1, most neck-pain sufferers need to practise regular cervical retractions. Research shows that a retraction program does not increase the range of neck movement so much as it relocates the resting position of the head to a better position above the shoulders. This neutral position minimizes tension on the small cervical muscles, and perhaps even on the local nerves.

Poor neck posture in sitting is almost universal. Most of today's workforce sits at computer terminals or spends the day looking down at work surfaces, moving belts, or machines. Changing your sitting posture is critical, and that change begins with correcting the curve in your lower back. Use a low back support or lumbar roll. I believe that the lumbar roll can be just as useful to patients with neck problems and cervicogenic headaches as it is to those with mechanical low back pain.

Whenever possible, put your computer screen or work surface at a level that allows you to maintain good upper back posture with your shoulders balanced and your neck retracted. As with any mechanical problem, try to change position as often as possible. No matter how good your posture may be, staying in one position too long will load that sore "thing" in your cervical spine until it starts to cause pain in your neck. That hurt may spread to your head.

### My therapist says she can help with laser therapy or a thing called TENS. What is it, and how does it work?

Transcutaneous electrical nerve stimulation (TENS) is intended to alter the body's ability to feel pain. Commercially available, externally applied electrical stimulation devices have been used in pain management for over a century. Presently, it is used almost exclusively by physiotherapists and chiropractors. A weak electrical current is applied to the skin and is presumed to pass through the tissues to reach the nerves. Combining a small additional current with the natural electrical flow within the nerves is thought to disrupt the transmission of pain. No one is sure exactly how it works and many researchers wonder whether it does anything at all. The results of treatment may show nothing more than the placebo effect. A placebo is a medication, treatment, or device that delivers no discernable benefit but nevertheless produces a favourable therapeutic response.

Cold laser therapy is based on properties of the laser beam that do not actually exist. The usefulness of this treatment, if any, should be considered a placebo effect.

Both of these treatments, and a wide range of other modalities are, at best, passive means of temporarily reducing the pain. They are little better than self-administered counterirritation. I will have more to say about this type of treatment in Chapter 11.

## If the goal of mechanical treatment is to restore movement, what about mobilization or cervical manipulation?

The terms mobilization and manipulation are used to describe two different aspects of manual or hands-on therapy. Mobilization refers to an applied movement where a joint or group of joints is moved passively to the limit of the normal range and then returned to the starting point. Manipulation refers to a manual technique where the joint is pushed slightly beyond the limit of its usual physiological range. Manipulation is frequently accompanied by that cracking noise often reported by patients undergoing chiropractic adjustments. *Adjustment* is the chiropractic term for manipulation.

If you are convinced that a cervicogenic headache is the result of tightness in a particular small cervical joint, then freeing the joint through mobilization or manipulation would make sense. But since the precise source of neck-related headaches has never been established, this is only speculation. Studies have found that both manipulation and mobilization may help, but the evidence is far from conclusive. In one study, simple massage worked as well as manipulation. As mentioned in Chapter 5, manual therapy on the cervical spine also carries with it a remote risk of serious vascular injury. Of greater importance in the treatment of headache is the fact that any excessive movement, either self-induced during a program of protraction, retraction, and nods, or through the hands of a therapist or chiropractor, can rapidly increase the pain.

## What about traction?

For neck-dominant pain, traction can be helpful but it is quite unpredictable. With headache, traction is not only unpredictable but is easily capable of aggravating the pain. In any case, most headache patients won't tolerate the traction halter.

## What about medication?

The idea that most cervicogenic headaches are mechanical suggests that, as in the treatment of neck and back pain, medication is a last resort. At this stage, I would use over-the-counter painkillers in preference to anything else, thought NSAIDs are frequently used, and have been reported to give some short-term relief. It is always a question of balancing the benefits of a medication against its potential risks and complications. With the exception of the routine use of narcotics, I have no objection to someone using most pain-relieving medications for a short period. And with a bad headache, that may be a sensible thing to do. I merely emphasize the fact that the source of the pain and many of its repercussions can be addressed more simply, economically, and, perhaps, more safely by non-medicinal means.

### So controlling mechanical headaches is really no different than controlling mechanical neck pain?

That's right. It's surprising how little it takes. Changing the way you sit behind the steering wheel may be enough. You can give yourself a headache from reading in bed. Not because the light is poor, but because it is almost impossible to get into a position that does not stress your neck. You could try something as elaborate as a reading stand or something as simple as sitting in a chair to read before you go to bed. I remember one patient who awoke every morning with severe headaches. It turned out she was sleeping on a solid, foam rubber pillow. The springy block created resistance against the weight of her head, and her neck muscles tightened in response. The action of stabilizing her neck all night made her muscles sore and that developed into her headache. That was a long time ago, and ever since I have suggested that patients with cervicogenic headaches never use a solid foam rubber pillow. It's like that bad joke about the restless sleeper with the rubber pillow who erased his head. Only the real result, a headache, isn't at all amusing.

You can get a headache from treating your low back. I tried to help a neighbour of mine with her Pattern 1 low back pain. My strategy included teaching her to do frequent repetitions of the sloppy push-up. Treating friends is always problematic because they are not really patients, so I tend to be less detailed in my instructions and less meticulous in my follow-up. I left my neighbour with a set of instructions and went on my way. The next I heard about her back pain was from her husband. I asked him how she was doing and he told me that she had stopped my exercises because they gave her terrible headaches. The headaches were far worse than her back pain had ever been. She didn't want to tell me because I was, after all, a friend. I knew the source of the headaches immediately. The sloppy push-up requires you to raise your upper body. If your technique is not right, you tend to use your neck muscle to assist your arms. This causes your neck to arch and tightens the muscles at the base of the skull. And so the headache begins. Two patients out of every ten who begin doing sloppy push-ups for Pattern 1 low back pain develop headaches. Correcting the exercise technique eliminates the problem. I make a point of cautioning my patients about this complication. Unfortunately for my friend, she was in my neighbourhood and not in my practice.

When I started to scuba dive, I used to come out of the water after every session with a nasty headache. I assumed the pain was the result of the difference in air pressure under the water and at the surface. I suspected that I was not equalizing my ear pressure adequately. But then I noticed that if I watched the bottom while I was diving and didn't try to look up, my headache wasn't so bad. I realized that it was not my ears or the atmosphere, but my scuba gear, that was to blame. I was wearing an old-style buoyancy compensator that fit around the neck like a yoke on an ox. It pulled down on my cervical spine and forced me to strain against it whenever I tried to look up. I changed to an inflatable vest and my headaches disappeared.

Making simple changes in your everyday activities can have significant benefit. Controlling your headache will let you continue to do whatever you want to do.

# CHAPTER SEVEN

## *Big, Scary Words*

I don't think there is a greater barrier to understanding or coping with back and neck pain than the terminology that doctors, physiotherapists, and chiropractors use to describe ordinary mechanical problems. Some of it constitutes professional jargon, a form of streamlined communication that allows medical professionals to discuss complicated issues in a quick and efficient fashion. One example I frequently cite is the word "medial" – a word I use in my medical practice dozens of times every day. It means "nearer the median plane or axis of a body or part." In other words, it is the part closest to the centre. The medial side of your knee is the side that is next to your other leg. Try to think of another word in English that means exactly the same thing. There isn't one. But as convenient as the terminology may be within my profession, it is of no value if the person to whom I am speaking cannot speak my language.

Sometimes a word in medical jargon carries a different meaning than it does in ordinary conversation. "Acute" is an excellent example. When used by a physician to describe symptoms, "acute" refers only to timing. An acute onset is one that starts quickly. An acute episode is one that lasts for a short time. Back pain that lasts about six weeks is considered acute. Any back pain that lasts longer is termed sub-acute or chronic. The medical definition doesn't include the quality of the pain. But in everyday usage, acute generally refers to intensity. An acute pain is a severe pain. Some doctors use the word both ways. No wonder everyone get confused.

Many technical terms are built upon Greek or Latin roots with beginnings and endings that neatly include additional information. The ending "itis," for example, indicates the presence of inflammation – the redness, heat, and swelling that accompanies mechanical, chemical, or infective irritation. Words with "itis" endings have crept into common usage. Weekend athletes experience tendonitis or bursitis. Everyone has known the discomfort of pharyngitis (sore throat) or gastritis (stomach ache). Yet when "itis" is attached to words related to the spine, like arthritis or spondylitis, it seems so much more ominous.

Other expressions we commonly use reflect poorly conceived attempts to translate medical reality into popular culture. One of the most troubling is the "slipped disc." Discs narrow, bulge, dry out, fissure, and even rupture, but they never slip! The mental picture created by this inaccurate term is far more frightening than the real physical problem. Can you imagine the chaos if your discs really could pop out of your spine at the least provocation? Many people think it actually happens. They see their spine coming uncoupled or collapsing like a house of cards. The apprehension created by that false image prevents them from trying active treatment or living a full life.

### If my disc can't slip, can it disintegrate?

That is another term that makes the disc sound very fragile. The vision of disintegrating discs in your neck might have you waiting for your head to disconnect and fall off. It never will. Discs dry out as we grow older; the chemical composition does change. The centre of the disc loses its elasticity and becomes more fibrous and gristly. It can even dry to the point where there are open gas-filled spaces. The shell of the disc ages too. It becomes less resilient and elastic. Disc height can narrow from a couple of centimetres down to a few millimetres. But it never disintegrates.

## What does my doctor mean when he says I have degenerative disc disease?

Degeneration is a term with variable meanings. Applied to a disc, it generally denotes the normal ageing process I have just described. In our teenage years, the discs are 90 per cent water, but by the age of sixty, the water content is down to 60 per cent and still falling. That is not a disease process, though, unless you consider age a disease. I admit it does have several of the characteristics of illness. But labelling the ageing back as having degenerative disc disease (DDD) not only sounds frightening, it implies that some day there will be a cure for the problem. This creates an expectation and attitude in the patient that may cause him or her to resist committing to a lifetime program of management and control.

And while we are talking about discs, I should clear up the confusion about "bulging" discs. As the disc dries, the outer shell fails, and material from the inside can push outward through a crack. The bulge on the disc may be called a rupture, herniation, protrusion, disruption, or, if the bump separates from the shell, a sequestration. All the words refer to the same thing: a failure of the outer shell. If that bump hits a nerve, some doctors refer to it inaccurately as an "acute disc." I don't know why they would consider a bump that touches a nerve more acute than one that doesn't. In that instance, it is the nerve that has been suddenly affected, not the disc. It should be called an "acute nerve."

## You said discs weren't fragile. Why do I hear of so many people whose backs go out?

I have always wanted to see a back "go out." I joke with patients that if I could watch their back go out, I would probably know where it went. Then I could retrieve it and make it "go in." The expression, of course, refers to the sudden onset of back pain accompanied by that dramatic body shift to one side that many people experience. It certainly feels as if part of the back has gone out of place, but this is not what happens. The pain originates in the discs, joints, or ligaments, and initiates the muscle response that creates the shift. But the shift takes place without disrupting the normal connections between the adjacent bones.

If there is an expression that intrigues me even more than the back "going out," it is when someone says, "I've thrown my back out." Now there's a daunting prospect: living without a spine, and with the personal responsibility for having done such a stupid thing. Fortunately, backs cannot be thrown out, nor do they ever choose to leave on their own.

### I have a friend who was told she has arthritis in her spine. Isn't that serious?

Arthritis is a very non-specific word. The first part, "arth," comes from the Latin for joint. The "itis" means inflammation. Put together, the word means inflammation in a joint, but it says nothing about the cause or how serious the condition might be.

If I accidentally pinched the end of my finger in the door and the joint at the end of my finger became swollen and inflamed, I would now technically qualify as an arthritis sufferer. Never mind that there was no permanent damage done, bone broken, or danger of ongoing problems.

### But that's silly! What you have is a sore finger, not arthritis.

That's my point. The word *arthritis* does not distinguish between a serious or permanent illness and a temporary minor injury. All it says is that a joint somewhere in the body is inflamed for some time for any reason. Pattern 2 back pain probably arises in small spinal joints that are irritated and worn due to constant use and normal ageing. That irritation may well lead to inflammation, and that inflammation in the small facet joints of the spine can correctly be labelled arthritis. But it is not a disease and it is not permanent.

### One of my friends has rheumatoid arthritis. Is that the same thing?

The term rheumatoid arthritis has two parts. Arthritis means an inflamed joint. Rheumatoid is the name of a systemic disease that can contribute to that inflammation. In rheumatoid disease, the body appears to react against itself as if it were fighting a foreign invader. This process can affect many systems, including the skin, the internal organs, the nerves, and, of course, the joints. Although it affects less than 3 per cent of the population, rheumatoid disease in its most severe form can cause significant and permanent joint destruction. But keep that in perspective. Less than 2 per cent of the population have the full-blown disease and only 10 per cent of those people have severe joint problems.

According to the American Rheumatism Association, 25 per cent of patients with rheumatoid arthritis recover normal joint function completely and another 25 per cent experience complete healing with only minor residual deformities. Still, the spectre of rheumatoid disease creates the fear that haunts the word arthritis. Ironically, some doctors use the diagnosis "a touch of arthritis," intending to reassure patients with minor mechanical back pain. To the uninformed, however, the word arthritis summons up a vision of life in a wheelchair with deformed hands, feet, and knees. Hardly reassuring, is it?

### Can rheumatoid arthritis affect the joints of the spine as well?

Yes, it can, particularly the joint between C1 and C2. The ligaments that bind the peg of C2 to the ring of C1 loosen as a result of the chronic inflammation. This allows C1 to slip forward on top of C2. The spinal cord that runs through the canal behind the peg is obviously at risk. This high in the spine, cord damage can be catastrophic. It is a serious complication of rheumatoid disease, and one that requires aggressive medical attention that may include surgery.

### Is osteoarthritis the same thing?

No. Osteoarthritis refers to the type of inflammation that can be caused just by natural ageing. The same process occurs following a joint injury, where the joint wears out prematurely. Although osteoarthritis is perhaps the correct term to use when discussing certain types of mechanical back pain, I find it more comfortable to talk about advancing maturity, wear and tear, or the normal effects of age than about degenerative discs and osteoarthritic joints.

**My sister was told that she had a slip in her low back. The doctor showed her an X-ray where the bones were out of place. But if discs don't slip, how can that be?**

Discs in your back never slip, but sometimes the bones do move. The condition is called spondylolisthesis. The first part, "spondyl," refers to the spine. Anything relating to the spine may have "spondyl" in its name. The last part, "listhesis," means slip. In plain language, spondylolisthesis means a slip in the spine.

This is not a rare condition and it often goes undetected throughout life. Occasionally it is first noticed in late adolescence when it is associated with severe back pain and spasm in the hamstring muscles. More often, it is

### Degenerative Spondylolisthesis

*Degenerative spondylolisthesis is produced when the interlocking facet joints wear down and partially lose contact. Because the roof of the spinal canal remains intact, this type of slip decreases the canal size and can cause Pattern 4 pain.*

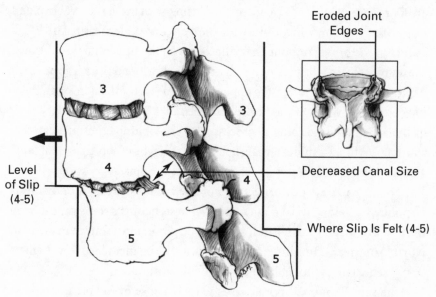

found by chance in adults when the back is X-rayed for some other reason. The slip is not always painful and, as you grow older, the slip itself is increasingly unlikely to be a significant cause of back pain.

Bones may slip out of alignment for various reasons, everything from certain types of bone disease to a major injury. But there are two types of spondylolisthesis that we see most often. The first occurs in women more often than men, and generally appears at age forty or later. The slip typically takes place between L4 and L5 (the second-last and last moving segments in the lumbar spine) and is associated with wearing out of the interlocking facet joints. These joints are normally L shaped but are flattened by wear. As they flatten, they allow one vertebra to slide over the other. The mechanical failure can cause Pattern 1 or 2 back-dominant pain, and the associated narrowing of the spinal canal is one of the recognized causes of Pattern 4 leg-dominant pain.

The other type of slip occurs with equal frequency in both sexes, and generally occurs between L5 and S1, the next level down. This slip is initiated by a break in the posterior wall of the spinal canal. On the back of the canal there are four joints: two at the upper end, which link with the vertebra above, and two at the bottom, which join with the vertebra underneath. The break occurs in the bridge of bone that runs between the upper and lower pairs. The joints remain attached to the adjacent vertebra, but pull apart from each other. Without that contact, the upper joints slide forward, taking with them the body of the vertebra and the front of the canal. The lower joints, the back of the canal, and the spinous process (the bony bumps that you can feel running down your spine) remain behind. In this type of slip, the spinal canal actually enlarges, so there is less chance of nerve compression.

A break in those posterior parts of the spine is called spondylolysis ("spondyl" = spine, "lysis" = cut). Spondylolysis happens some time during the first five years or so of life. It seems to be present in about 10 per cent of North Americans. In some Inuit populations, the incidence is as high as 50 per cent. This is probably a genetic predisposition.

When the slip of the bones takes place because of the break between the upper and lower joints, the condition goes by the majestic name of spondylitic (or lytic) spondylolisthesis.

## Lytic Spondylolisthesis

*Lytic spondylolisthesis results from breaks in the bridges of bone joining the upper and lower facets. As the slip progresses and the gap widens, the spinous process and the inferior facet are left behind and the size of the spinal canal increases.*

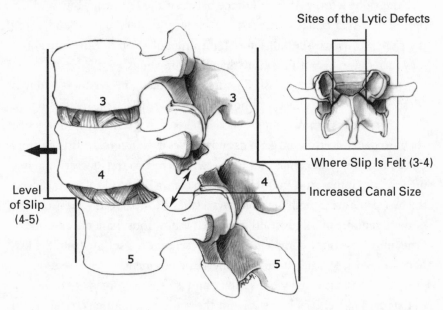

## If someone told me I had that, I would be terrified. Do the medical terms have to sound so frightening?

The names aren't frightening if you know what they mean. They are simply a convenient way for doctors to exchange information. Saying "spondylitic spondylolisthesis" is considerably faster than saying "a condition of the back where the superior vertebra slides forward on the inferior vertebra as a result of a long-standing defect in the posterior elements of the vertebral structure at the pars interarticularis between the superior and inferior zygoapophyseal joints." If you were the doctor, which description would you choose?

But I agree that many of the terms doctors use can and should be simplified. One of my favourite examples is the diagnosis of cervical spondylosis. "Cervical" means neck and "spondyl" means spine. The ending "osis" just means "a problem with." So cervical spondylosis means "you've got something wrong with your neck." Not much insight provided, but it's quick and sounds impressive.

Mark Twain once said, "The difference between the almost right word and the right word is the difference between the lightning-bug and the lightning." As a back- or neck-pain patient, understanding and using the right words is essential. Those lightning bolts you're worrying about may turn out to be nothing more than lightning bugs.

One technical term I wish doctors and patients understood better is "dysaesthesia." "Dys" means abnormal and "aesthesia" means feeling. In English, it means funny feelings. Dysaesthesia is that weird sensation when your arm falls asleep or you get pins and needles in your foot. It also describes that strange impression that your limb is wrapped in cotton or wearing a sock or glove. Paraesthesia means the same thing ("para" = outside of normal), and the two terms are interchangeable. Dysaesthesia (or paraesthesia) is not the same as genuine numbness, although that is how most patients describe it. True numbness is the complete absence of sensation resulting from the loss of nerve signal, typically from direct nerve involvement.

Dysaesthesia is usually not serious, and is caused by message overload, not signal failure. It is like static on the radio when an electrical storm is near. The station is transmitting and your radio is receiving, but you can't hear the music for all that crackling. Interference with the regular nerve signal can arise from both mechanical Patterns 1 and 2 and from Pattern 4. Of course, it can also accompany the pinched nerve of Pattern 3.

One patient of mine is a good example. She found that her left leg would "go numb" every time she walked down a steep hill. She had no leg pain, just "numbness." When she climbed the hill, the leg would always feel normal. I questioned her about the numbness. She said her leg wasn't exactly numb; it just felt like it had gone to sleep with pins and needles everywhere. The examination showed no sign of nerve irritation and the tests for power, reflex, and sensation were all normal. What produced her problem? Her posture. When she walked down the hill, she arched her back and irritated her small spinal joints. The extra neural input through branches of the nerves to her leg started the "crackling" she felt as pins and needles. When she was on her way up the hill, she bent forward and took the strain off the facet joints. No strain meant no extra input, and therefore no dysaesthesia. She never had a pinched nerve.

**I understand that most spine pain is mechanical and harmless, but there must be more serious causes. What are they?**
A large number of conditions unrelated to the spine can cause back or neck pain. The tearing of the inner wall of the great blood vessel from the heart, the aorta, can be felt as a searing pain in the back. Gall bladder disease can sometimes cause back pain, and so can a kidney stone. Here is a list of some of the more common or serious non-mechanical sources of back and neck pain. It's important to remember that everything in this list, and many other causes besides, account for less than 8 per cent of sore backs and necks.

### Ankylosing Spondylitis
The name describes an inflammation of the spine that leads to self-fusion. It is primarily a disease of young men and has very distinctive characteristics. They include a visible flattening of the surface of the low back, loss of chest movement, and progressive stiffness in the joints along the spine. About half of the cases have significant stiffness in the hips and knees as well. The spinal stiffness is particularly noticeable first thing in the morning and is greatly relieved by exercise or physical activity. The disease generally begins in the low back and, as it progresses upward, it stiffens the back by fusing the vertebrae together. Ankylosing spondylitis may subside and the progression will stop.

Because much of the inflammation and pain is in the spinal joints, patients find it most comfortable to bend forward. Unfortunately, this often becomes the posture in which their spines fuse. In the rare, extreme case when the fusion process reaches the neck, patients may find it impossible to raise their heads. They walk staring at the floor. This disease is not common, and even when it strikes, over 75 per cent of its victims continue to function normally. The diagnosis is made by physical examination, X-rays, and specific blood tests.

## Cancer

Primary cancer of the spine is rare. The most common types occur within the bone marrow in older patients. Malignant tumours can arise from any structure in the spine except the intervertebral disc. But except for the cancers of the bone-forming elements in the marrow, the incidence is extremely small.

Secondary or metastatic cancer of the spine is more common, but is still relatively infrequent. Secondary cancers originate somewhere else in the body and then spread to the spine. They most commonly affect the thoracic spine and are least common in the neck. Metastatic tumours tend to affect the vertebral bodies more than the posterior elements. One of the hallmarks of spine cancer is a history of unremitting non-mechanical pain that is unaffected by movement or position. The sites of the original tumours in decreasing order of frequency are breast (for women only), lung, prostate, kidney, and stomach. Having a cancer somewhere else in the body does not always mean that new back or neck pain signals metastatic spread. This possibility must be considered, but it may well be that the spine pain is nothing more than a simple mechanical problem unrelated to the cancer.

## Klippel-Feil Syndrome

The Klippel-Feil Syndrome and its associated abnormalities are a group of birth defects in the cervical spine. The most visible features are a short neck and restricted neck movement. There is sometimes an elevation of one or both shoulder blades and a webbing of the skin from the shoulders to below the ears. Because the spinal defect is part of a more widespread problem, there are a number of other associated abnormalities involving the central nervous system, the urinary system, and the cardiovascular system. Like many congenital problems, the severity varies widely from case to case. Some children have only a spontaneous fusion of one or more of their upper cervical vertebrae, which produces a modest loss of normal movement. The majority of affected individuals lead normal lives.

## Paget's Disease

Normal bones are constantly replaced as new material is laid down and the old material is removed and recycled. In Paget's disease, this balance is disrupted. The old bone is not removed adequately and the new bone is of poor quality. The bones become misshapen and have a brittle, chalky character. Pain may arise from the bones themselves, or from pressure on the spinal cord or a nerve root caused by the altered contour of the vertebrae. Over time, the abnormal bone growth results in a typical short stature and forward-bent posture.

## Scheuermann's Disease

This abnormality is also called juvenile round back. The problem occurs within the growth plates of the vertebral bodies. As they enlarge, they do not produce the normal drum shape, but create a forward-facing wedge instead. By definition, Scheuermann's disease applies only to spines where the growth abnormality occurs in three adjacent bones. The condition typically occurs in the thoracic spine, where the stack of wedges creates an increased forward curve, or thoracic kyphosis. There is a large natural variation in the normal amount of forward curve in this part of the spine. Not everyone with poor posture has Scheuermann's disease. Usually only forward curves over forty-five degrees are considered for treatment.

## Spina Bifida

I've included spina bifida in this list only because so many people wrongly believe that because it occurs in the spine, it must be a cause of back pain. This condition exhibits a huge range of severities. The worst situation is a devastating condition called meningomyelocoele, which occurs when the spinal canal completely fails to close during foetal development. The nerves that would normally be within the spinal canal are contained instead in a large pouch on the infant's back. In the most extreme form, the underdeveloped spine contains no neural elements at all and there is complete paralysis below the defect. Fortunately, this extreme abnormality is very rare, but minor variations do occur.

During foetal growth, the tube of the spinal canal is formed from front to back. The sides of the canal grow from the back of the vertebral body, arching together until they meet in the middle to close the tube. Then the growth extends back further to form the spinous process. Failure to close the canal completely means there will be no spinous process, and a small gap (usually one to two millimetres) will exist between the two sides of the canal. This narrow space is filled with strong fibrous tissue. Secure within the virtually complete canal, the nerves function normally. Because the bony defect has no relation to the interlocking facet joints, there is no possibility for slip or any increase in the risk of back pain. Because this tiny defect cannot be detected on physical examination and is frequently overlooked on X-ray, the condition is often called spina bifida occulta (occulta meaning "hidden"). Spina bifida occulta in the adult spine is of no clinical significance and does not cause pain.

### You didn't mention scoliosis. Isn't that a serious disease?

Scoliosis is not a disease but a description of the shape of the spine. When viewed from the side, the normal back has three curves: lordosis in the neck and low back and kyphosis in between. Seen from front to back, the normal spine is a straight line. Scoliosis is a side-to-side curve. The scoliotic spine also tends to rotate so some ribs or the hip may push forward more on one side and fall back on the other side. Abnormal curvature affects about 4 per cent of the population, but the incidence increases in the older age groups. Some studies suggest 15 per cent of people over age sixty have a side-to-side curvature.

By far the most common type of scoliosis is idiopathic. The name means "without cause." Idiopathic scoliosis occurs more in girls than boys and typically first appears between the ages of nine and thirteen. It is often first recognized by body asymmetry, a low shoulder, a prominent ribcage, or a protruding hip. The diagnosis is frequently made by a gym teacher, school nurse, or even a friend.

Most idiopathic curves are mild and require no treatment. The curvature will progress only until the end of skeletal growth, on average around age sixteen, and will then remain unchanged through adult life.

## Does scoliosis hurt?

Minor curves are pain-free and the chance of having back pain with scoliosis is about the same as for the rest of us. When pain does occur, it is still in a typical mechanical fashion, with Pattern 1 being more frequent than Pattern 2.

As the amount of curve increases, there is an increase in the frequency of pain. Back pain is more frequent when the curve is primarily in the lower spine. Thoracic scoliosis is more common, but more often remains pain-free.

## When should scoliosis be treated?

The girl with idiopathic scoliosis usually has a curve in her upper back pointing to the right and curved to the left. The associated rotation pushes ribs backward on the right and forward on the left. There is a compensating curve in the low back. When the curves balance, both the hips and the shoulders remain parallel to the floor. Curves measuring less than forty degrees on X-ray do not need to be treated.

During the period of spinal growth, some curves progress quite rapidly. For this reason, regular medical review is strongly recommended during puberty. Bracing may prevent curve progression in a girl who has not started her menstrual cycle or a boy who has not finished his adolescent growth spurt. After the end of growth, any correction of the scoliosis will require spinal surgery. Bracing, exercise, or spinal adjustment in the adult has no effect.

Even curves over forty degrees may require no treatment if they are well-balanced. Some people with scoliosis develop two primary curves: one in the chest and another curving in the opposite direction in the low back. These two curves may be so well-balanced that they cannot be detected when the person wears loose clothing. Although there will be a loss of height, when she is fully dressed her overall appearance is normal. Surgery need not be considered.

It is not always the amount of the curve that prompts the surgeon to act. Often, the severity of rotation and the size of rib hump at the back are the most cosmetically obvious abnormalities. Correcting that hump sometimes requires a separate operation, but the results can be remarkably good.

### You said there were other types of scoliosis?

In children, spinal curvature can be associated with a misshapen vertebra, a form of congenital abnormality. Curvature will also result if there is childhood paralysis, such as that associated with meningomyelocoele.

### You said that the incidence of scoliosis increases in older people. Why is that?

The rapid growth-related increase in the amount of the curve ends when spinal growth is finished. But it can still increase about one degree per year as the spine ages. As the discs dry and narrow, shortening the spine, it may not compress in a straight line. A minor pre-existing curve will become accentuated and may reach an angle that requires treatment. Even a straight spine may collapse into a curve, a condition called degenerative collapsing scoliosis.

Patients with degenerative scoliosis may exhibit the back-dominant symptoms of Patterns 1 and 2, and may develop the typical leg pain of Pattern 4, as well. The combination can be extremely disabling and, in some cases, serious enough to consider surgery.

### When would you recommend surgery for someone with degenerative collapsing scoliosis?

Sometimes the collapse stabilizes itself and sometimes it progresses so slowly that it never becomes a problem. I remember one patient, an avid golfer, who saw me for mechanical back pain from degenerative scoliosis. I recommended a program based on his pattern of pain and started him on a regular routine of trunk-strengthening exercises. I saw him every six months for the next ten years. He was able to control his pain but, more importantly for him, he continued to golf. As his scoliosis progressed, he became steadily shorter, until finally his ribs were resting on the top of his pelvis. Eventually he lost pain control and was forced to reduce the number of holes he played every week. That was the last straw. After more than a decade of success with conservative care, I finally operated to stabilize his spine and regain some of his lost height. The operation was successful and he is golfing again.

## Does the collapse of the spine in the older patient have anything to do with osteoporosis?

Osteoporosis describes a natural thinning of the bones. It is an unavoidable part of growing older. The normal process of replenishing healthy bone falls out of balance, and the elements that remove the bone proceed more rapidly than those that replace it. Two different kinds of cells are involved. One type, the osteoblast, generates new bone, while the other type, the osteoclast, removes and recycles material that's worn down, worn out, or damaged. This process allows the body to grow bone spurs or reshape the spinal joints and spinal canal to accommodate the changes of ageing. It is estimated that full replacement of a normal long bone in the average young adult takes about seven years.

Of course, there has to be a balance between the process of tearing down and building up. Certain hormones must be present to regulate the cells that carry out the repairs and replacements. In their younger years, most people maintain the proper balance between making and removing bone. But as they grow older, the process falters because of a hormonal imbalance, or for other reasons, such as deficiency of bone-forming materials. Bone creation slows down while bone destruction continues, perhaps even speeds up. The bones get thinner.

It's this imbalance that gets you into trouble. The bone that remains is normal. There is just less of it, and it is not as strong as it was. The outer shell of the bone, the cortex, becomes thinner, and the spongy bone inside changes significantly. Normally, the interior bone is made up of a number of adjacent cells, like rooms in a row. As osteoporosis advances, the walls of the rooms thin and some of them disappear, leaving the ceiling unsupported for longer and longer stretches. Not only is there less bone, but the structure of the bone that remains is less able to withstand the loads of your everyday activities. The interior spongy bone, called cancellous bone, makes up most of the vertebral body. This is one reason why the spine is so susceptible to the process of osteoporosis.

## Does osteoporosis hurt?

Not as long as the bone remains intact. But like a strand of rope whose fibres slowly fray and divide, there will come a time when the load will be too much and something will have to give.

While the presence of osteoporosis may be particularly obvious in the vertebrae, it can affect other bones as well. The wall of a normal eighty-year-old's thigh bone is 50 per cent thinner than it was at age thirty. The outside diameter of the bone remains the same, but the thickness of the wall is reduced from the inside, just the opposite of how a tree grows by adding an outside ring of wood year after year.

If you're over forty, some of the bones in your body may already have walls that are thinner than they once were. The walls are thickest when you are in your late twenties or early thirties. Much of the interior cancellous bone that is lost is replaced with fat.

## When the bone gives way, that's when osteoporosis becomes painful, right?

Osteoporosis itself never actually hurts, but a crushed vertebra certainly does. Although the fracture occurs because the bone is so frail, rather than breaking in a major injury, it is still a fracture, and that is very painful.

The stress required to fracture a vertebra in someone with advanced osteoporosis may be as little as a cough, a sneeze, or just stepping down off a curb. The bones have become fractures waiting to happen. And it is not only the spine that can crush or give way. In elderly patients, osteoporosis is a major predisposing factor in fractures of the hip and wrist. Both areas have large amounts of cancellous bone and relatively thin outer shells.

## What happens now?

Because the fracture occurs in a normal fashion, albeit through very thin bone, the healing proceeds in a normal fashion, as well. Cancellous bone takes about six weeks to heal, and although the pain can be severe during the first week or two, it generally subsides. Often, no treatment is necessary except for rest and protection, and, of course, adequate pain medication.

Once the vertebra collapses, it cannot return to its normal height. It heals in a new shape, a forward-facing wedge similar in shape to the ones described in Scheuermann's disease. When several of these crushed vertebrae are stacked together in the upper back, they produce a typical round-back deformity termed a dowager's hump.

Once the vertebra heals, most of the pain disappears. There may be some residual problems related to the new shape of the spine and the additional load placed on adjacent discs or joints. In rare cases, the bone fails to heal properly and the back pain persists. Treatment for that problem is one of the recent advances in spine surgery that I will discuss in Chapter 12.

### Exactly what causes osteoporosis?

Osteoporosis is a failure to balance bone turnover. No one knows why the failure occurs or why it is more pronounced in some individuals. We are all potentially at risk, because bone loss occurs in all of us, but there are definite risk factors. Osteoporosis is more common in women, affecting one woman in every three compared to one man in a dozen. Among women, the risk is higher for those who have had an early menopause or an early hysterectomy with removal of both ovaries, and for women missing periods for six months or longer (excluding pregnancy) as a result of over-exercising or over-dieting.

For both men and women, the risk of extensive osteoporosis is increased with the long-term use of high-dose steroids; a history of osteoporosis in either parent; medical conditions such as Cushing's syndrome, or thyroid diseases that retard bone formation or accelerate bone removal; malabsorption problems, such as Crohn's disease, that prevent nutrient uptake; long-term immobility; and heavy drinking or smoking. Even one or two of these factors increases your risk for developing clinically significant osteoporosis.

### Why would women have a higher risk for osteoporosis than men?

Part of the answer is the different hormonal arrangement of the female body. Osteoporosis is most aggressive after menopause or total hysterectomy, when the estrogen levels fall dramatically. Men never undergo a similar drastic shift in their hormone balance.

There is also a question of bone mass. Most research indicates that, in proportion to body weight, a typical woman has about 30 per cent less bone mass than a typical man. If a man and woman both experience the natural thinning of the bones at the same rate, the woman would suffer the consequences 30 per cent sooner.

And there are other, not-yet-understood factors. For instance, an accelerated form of osteoporosis affects white women more than those of other races.

### If osteoporosis doesn't hurt, how can I tell I have it before I break a bone?

First, review the list of risk factors. If you are a twenty-six-year-old man who doesn't smoke, drink, or have medical problems that interfere with bone formation, and your parents are healthy, you needn't worry and should not bother being investigated. If, however, you possess a few of the risk factors, and particularly if you are a post-menopausal woman, then it is a good idea to check it out. The best current technique for determining your degree of osteoporosis is to measure your bone density. The procedure is dual-energy X-ray absorptometry or a DEXA scan. The scan will produce pictures of your bones. It generally scans the most vulnerable areas: your back, your hips, and your wrists. You will usually get a computer printout describing your degree of osteoporosis relative to normal values for your age group. Not everyone needs a DEXA scan, but if you are in a high-risk group, ask your doctor to arrange one for you.

### What is the best treatment for osteoporosis?

As the cliché says, the best treatment is prevention. Although we have come a long way in managing fully established osteoporosis, you are still far better off if you can avoid the problem in the first place. Developing strong bones is something you must begin in your teens. It is frightening to think that in North America today, experts estimate that less than 25 per cent of the young women are taking in enough calcium to allow adequate bone growth. Bones grow denser only in the first three decades of your life and by the time you are thirty, your bones are as strong as they will ever be. During your teens and twenties, adequate bone growth requires at least 1,300 milligrams of elemental calcium a day, combined with about 400 units of vitamin D.

If you are a woman, you should maintain a regular daily intake of approximately 1,000 milligrams of elemental calcium until menopause. After that, increase the amount to between 1,200 and 1,500 milligrams daily. Men should take at least 1,000 milligrams of calcium a day as well.

Dietary calcium can be obtained from dairy products, including cheese and yogourt. It is also available from leafy vegetables, baked beans, egg yolks, liver, salt-water or bony fish, dried fruit, and fortified juices. A lot of older people, and anyone who is lactose-intolerant, cannot use dairy products to meet the calcium requirements. An alternative is to take a calcium supplement, and there is a wide variety available. However you take it, maintaining an adequate calcium intake is essential.

### I understand that diet is important. What else can I do?

The guidelines for minimizing osteoporosis reflect the risk factors. If you are a smoker, stop smoking. If you drink alcohol, do so in moderation. Do weight-bearing exercises regularly; they help maintain bone density. Your bones and muscles are very responsive to the demands you place upon them. The more you use them, the stronger they remain. One study has shown that strong muscles along the spine can reduce the incidence of vertebral fractures in women with established osteoporosis.

### Is medication helpful?

Currently, the most promising drugs for the prevention and even treatment of osteoporosis are the bisphosphonates. This class of drugs acts to reduce the rate of bone loss. Most of the bisphosphonates can be taken orally, although some require regular injections. They are effective only when taken with adequate amounts of calcium and vitamin D.

## Isn't hormone replacement supposed to help too?

Estrogen, the hormone the bones are missing, is typically prescribed in combination with a progestin and has been used for decades to prevent bone loss in post-menopausal women. These same two hormones are used in birth-control pills. The hormones are usually taken in monthly cycles and may restart menstruation in a post-menopausal patient. This is just one of the many potential complications from using these powerful agents.

## What other side effects can occur?

Studies have shown that women taking an estrogen/progestin combination have a relatively increased risk factor for heart disease, invasive breast cancer, stroke, and pulmonary embolism. This list of possible complications must be balanced against the potential benefits. With osteoporosis, the benefit is a suspension or reversal of declining bone density. A recent clinical study was abruptly ended when it was established that although the risk factors for hip fracture were decreased by 34 per cent, the increased relative risk factor for all the complications was considerably higher. That makes it sound like hormone therapy can be very dangerous. But the situation is not quite so clear-cut. Be careful how you read the numbers. The increase in the absolute risks of heart disease, breast cancer, stroke, and pulmonary embolism were exceedingly modest; seven or eight cases per ten thousand person-years of estrogen/progestin use. Looking at the number of actual cases, the danger doesn't seem as great. The study looked at the safety and value of hormone-replacement therapy for post-menopausal women. But it cannot answer the question, "Is the risk worth the benefits?" Each woman must evaluate her own situation with her physician.

## Then what do you say to a patient who is already taking hormone-replacement therapy or who wants to start?

I explain the pros and cons of the treatment and emphasize that it is a serious decision that should not be taken lightly or hastily. In addition to understanding her specific risks and benefits, each woman must also realize that once the estrogen/progestin replacement is stopped, the bone loss will rapidly return to its normal rate. She will be no further ahead. If she took the hormones for two years after menopause and then stopped, her chance of developing osteoporosis from then on would the same as if she had never taken hormone replacement at all. Selecting this form of osteoporosis control is never an easy decision.

### Are there any other options?

There is a class of related drugs called selective estrogen receptor modulators, or SERMs. They appear to act like estrogen without targeting the breast and cardiac tissue. They have been reported to reduce the number of fractures in the spine. These drugs are approved for use in Canada but are relatively new and have not yet undergone the type of extensive clinical trials that raised doubts about the use of hormone-replacement therapy.

### Maybe I should just give up smoking, limit my drinking, and stay with calcium replacement and exercise?

Those are excellent choices in any case. Adding medication or hormone replacement may help, but the best strategy is still to maximize your bone mass when you are young and protect it as you grow older.

There is one small caution about exercise. We know that your bones respond to regular activity and there are studies that suggest women who exercise regularly seem to lose less calcium than those who don't exercise at all. But there is also evidence that extremely strenuous workouts can upset the hormonal balance. Doctors have found that female athletes who run more than thirty-two kilometres (twenty miles) per week may develop amenorrhea, where the menstrual cycle stops. The theory is that when body fat drops below a certain critical level, estrogen production also drops. The presence of amenorrhea is a clear indication that the hormones are askew, and the low estrogen predisposes to rapid osteoporosis. A woman of twenty-five who exercises excessively (training at an Olympic level) may suffer as much bone loss as an average woman would expect at age fifty.

**I don't think exercising at that level is something I'll have to worry about.**

I agree that for most of us that won't be the problem. Dealing with osteoporosis in particular is very much like dealing with neck and back pain in general. Use moderation, develop healthy habits, and take control of your own situation.

**I can't control the situation if somebody smashes into the back of my car and gives me whiplash. That's not my fault.**

Maybe not. But before we get into that, there's a more important medical issue. And it's this: you don't *have* whiplash. Whiplash is not an ailment or a physical injury. It merely describes the movement of your neck under certain specific conditions. That movement may or may not cause injury.

The commonest cause of the whiplash movement is the impact of one vehicle striking another from behind. The effect on your neck when you are in the car that is hit is not the same as what happens when you are in the car that delivers the blow. The forces involved are quite different and the impact throws you in distinctly opposite directions.

If your car strikes another or runs into a solid obstacle, your body will be restrained by your seat belt but your head will be thrown forward. It can't move very far before your chin hits your chest. That can hurt. It may bruise your chin and your chest and wrench the muscles in the back of your neck. But the distance your head can travel is limited. Because your neck is protected from further movement by the chin-chest contact, there is no whiplash effect.

Now consider what happens if you are in the car that gets rear-ended. When your vehicle is struck, it is suddenly pushed forward and your whole body goes with it except for your head. Unless your headrest is high enough (and it rarely is), there is nothing behind your head to support it or to carry it forward with your shoulders. It gets left behind as the car scoots forward beneath it. There is no equivalent at the back of your skull to your chin striking your chest, so your head snaps backward as far as the muscles, ligaments, and bones will allow. Some people recall their heads going back so far that they could see through the car's rear window. An instant after this violent backward motion, the elastic muscles and ligaments in your neck recoil and throw your head forward. This cycle can be repeated two or three times.

Your neck has experienced the movement called whiplash. Whether whiplash causes an injury or not depends on many things: the length and strength of your neck, the force of the impact, and the direction in which you were looking at the time of the accident, to name just a few.

### Will I always suffer that whiplash action if my car is struck from behind?

Not necessarily. If the impact is slight, there may be no neck movement at all. But a collision velocity of only twelve kilometres per hour (7.2 miles per hour) between vehicles of approximately the same size will produce that whiplash effect. That's one reason why a properly positioned headrest is as important to the protection of your spine as a properly applied seat belt and an air bag.

You might avoid whiplash if the back of your car seat is tipped back far enough. With enough slope, the forward movement of your car is translated into an upward movement of your body. A three-point belt restrains your hips and chest in the seat but allows your head to rise. Instead of the whiplash effect, your neck is stretched. Some people even report hitting the top of their head on the roof of the car. The mechanism is different, but you can still injure your spine.

### Is whiplash only associated with car accidents?

No, it isn't. The term whiplash was first used by an orthopaedic surgeon, H. E. Crowe, in 1928 to represent a specific movement. Anything that produced that movement could be considered whiplash. It was described, for example, in the pilots of airplanes that were catapulted from the deck of a ship (a practice that predated the modern aircraft carrier). Dr. Crowe clearly described whiplash as a mechanism, not as the injury or illness it came to represent.

Today's common belief that whiplash is an injury capable of causing a wide range of physical, neurological, and emotional problems was mirrored nearly 150 years ago by a malady called "railway spine." At that time, before modern equipment and safety standards, many people were seriously injured or killed in major rail accidents. Many others involved in minor mishaps appeared to have received no injury at all, yet went on to develop the same constellation of symptoms that are now associated with whiplash.

### So is whiplash real?

That simple question has produced fifty years of heated debate. We are not arguing with the reality of the mechanism. Everyone agrees that the neck can be flung back and forth. We are debating the effects of that motion, and whether or not it causes a specific injury.

Some believe that whiplash implies a frequent and potentially serious trauma. This group includes many personal-injury lawyers, who sue on their client's behalf to obtain financial compensation for extensive and permanent disabilities. Others believe that the whiplash injury does not exist. This group includes many insurance representatives, who regard the large claims for whiplash injury to be exaggerated, if not frankly fraudulent.

Like many medical practitioners, I tend to take a middle position. The mechanism of whiplash can certainly produce physical injury. In 1987, a group of medical doctors, chiropractors, physiotherapists, and bio-mechanical experts in Quebec prepared a classification of whiplash injuries. Their work coined the term whiplash-associated disorders (WAD) and their classification had four grades. Grade 0 implied no complaint about the neck and no physical signs. Grade 1 indicated a complaint of neck pain, stiffness, or tenderness only, with no objective findings. Grade 2 required complaints of neck pain, stiffness, or tenderness with physical changes, including a decreased range of movement and local tenderness. Grade 3 was the complaint of neck pain with evidence of a neurological injury such as loss of reflexes, muscle weakness, or altered sensation. The WAD Grade 4 was reserved for neck pain accompanied by X-rays showing a fracture or dislocation of the bones in the neck.

All four grades could include hearing loss, dizziness, a ringing in the ears, headache, poor memory, problems swallowing, and pain in the jaw joints. The Quebec Task Force, as it was called, recommended that patients with Grade 1 injuries return to their usual activities immediately. Grades 2 and 3 should return to a normal routine as soon as possible, typically within one week for Grade 2 and within three weeks for Grade 3. Grade 4 WAD, with recognized bony injuries, was treated on a case-by-case basis depending upon the severity of the fracture.

Overall, most patients with whiplash-related injuries made an excellent recovery when treated only with reassurance, prescribed activity, and simple pain management. The overwhelming majority was functioning normally within a month or two, and only a small percentage was still having trouble after one year. The patients in that small group utilized most of the medical resources and were involved in the largest legal settlements.

I find the WAD classification useful for several reasons. First, it gives some objectivity to the whole question of whiplash injury. Second, it supports the view that most soft-tissue injuries to the neck do recover with time, and that a permanent or serious disability is quite rare. Third, it provides a basis for treatment, and allows both the patient and doctor to recognize when the problem should be investigated more extensively or treated more aggressively.

### But I have heard so many stories about the terrible effects of a whiplash. Where do they all come from?

People who suffer a serious motor-vehicle accident often have a great deal of pain. When they believe that the accident was not their fault, that pain is reinforced by a justifiable anger at the circumstances or perhaps, more particularly, anger toward the person who injured them. Strong emotional reactions to the accident and to the pain are predictors of a slower recovery. The relationship between pain, emotion, and behaviour is a subject I look at in more detail in Chapter 10.

The presence of many whiplash effects also has a cultural bias. Some legal systems recognize whiplash as a specific physical injury and award substantial compensation to someone who has it. In other areas, having a whiplash, specifically in a motor-vehicle accident, is not considered significant. Predictably, the incidence of whiplash litigation in these regions is extremely low. In one famous European study, researchers found that the frequency of chronic neck pain was higher in a group of patients who had never had a motor-vehicle accident than in a group who had suffered a rear-end collision. Not surprisingly, the country in the study did not recognize whiplash as an entity, and there was no legal mechanism to obtain financial reward.

**You're saying that the lawyers are to blame?**
Not entirely, although taking your whiplash pain to court is certainly not a good way to eliminate your symptoms. There are other reasons you may worry unnecessarily about your injuries or focus on your pain. I remember seeing a woman for a medical legal opinion three years after she had been rear-ended. She told me that she had been taken directly from the scene of the accident to a small local hospital where a young doctor had examined her. He told her, and she quoted him exactly, that hers was "the worst whiplash I have ever seen." For all I know, it may have been the first whiplash he had ever seen, but as far as the patient was concerned, she knew she had a serious and permanent neck injury.

One of my secretaries was in an accident where her car was struck from behind. She came to work that afternoon complaining of a very sore neck. My examination showed some reduced range of movement and local tenderness, but nothing else. By the WAD classification she was a Grade 2. Although I was sympathetic to her pain, I realized two things. First, the office was busy and I needed her at her desk, but second, and more importantly, her recovery would be quicker if she maintained as normal a routine as possible and did not focus on her pain. She took time off every day for therapy to help reduce the discomfort, and I did my best to lighten the workload, but she stayed at her job. And she recovered quickly and completely. What disturbed me more than her obvious suffering was the fact that three of the insurance adjusters who talked with her stressed that her insurance policy entitled her to take time off work with full pay. They insisted that she stop work immediately and spend the next three months (the duration of her coverage) resting at home. I can't think of a better recipe for disaster.

**You must agree that the term whiplash sounds frightening!**
Yes, it does, and that is a big part of the problem. Lawyers seem to savour the sound of the word. I have to admit that "whiplash" sounds a lot more dramatic and damaging in court than "simple sprain," or "minor soft-tissue injury." The lawyer's job is to win a generous settlement. To do that, he or she must make you appear as crippled as possible. No judge or jury is likely to award a significant amount of money if you suddenly jump up and announce that your neck is fine and you are feeling great. So the lawyer has an obligation to focus on your limitations and your pain. But in convincing the court of how disabled you are, your lawyer may also convince you. At the very least, the litigation process will constantly remind you of your discomfort and limitations.

Unfortunately, there are many doctors who use the term whiplash inappropriately as well. I don't know whether they do it for simple convenience, dramatic effect, or so they can take credit for the almost inevitable spontaneous recovery. Whatever their motives, the label does their patients no good. You may experience whiplash, but you cannot "have" it. Most of the time that experience will leave you with nothing more than a pulled muscle or a minor sprain of one of your small neck joints.

**But you did say that sometimes whiplash can fracture or dislocate the bones in your neck. Isn't a broken neck very dangerous?**
People naturally fear a broken neck or a broken back. Disrupting the alignment of the spinal vertebrae can lead to serious nerve or spinal-cord injury and may result in permanent paralysis. But, for every major neurological injury, there are hundreds of cases where the spine sustains a fracture and still continues to function normally. The slight compression fracture of a vertebral body in osteoporosis is never associated with nerve injury.

It surprises people to learn that a broken neck is not necessarily fatal or even crippling. A "broken neck" can describe any fracture of a vertebra in your cervical spine. Sometimes a small fracture is caused when the bony attachment of a ligament in the neck tears loose. That's like taking off in your motorboat without casting off the line and pulling the cleat out of the dock. In the neck, the ligament injury may not be serious, and the fact that it has affected the bone can actually accelerate the rate of repair. In a funny way, you might be better off with that kind of "broken" neck.

### When would you operate on a broken neck?

Surgery may be required to fuse an unstable fracture that has allowed the bones to shift from their proper positions. Urgent surgery may be required if the fracture causes pressure on the spinal cord, causing a partial loss of function. Removing the compression quickly appears to promote better recovery. For those who suffer total paralysis, an emergency operation is not likely to change the outcome. Surgical stabilization of their spine may be needed later to maximize residual function.

Sometimes even a fracture with instability can be treated without an operation. The spine can be stabilized in a device called a halo vest, which is a metal "halo" screwed to the skull and supported by metal posts anchored to a brace that fits over the shoulders. The halo vest effectively prevents movement, something an ordinary cervical collar cannot do. Although it is cumbersome, it may be the best method of maintaining proper alignment while the fracture heals.

### So not all broken backs need surgery, and sometimes a broken back is not even a serious problem?

The seriousness of a spinal fracture can be difficult to determine. But those that are stable, in good position, and produce no nerve injury may require no specific treatment except pain pills, a little time off work, and perhaps a brace.

When nerves are damaged, the nature of the injury depends on the location of the fracture in the spine. Fractures in the low back below the point where the spinal cord ends cannot produce the same extensive paralysis as a fracture in the neck or thoracic spine. These may damage the cord.

The fracture type matters, as well. One type, aptly named a "burst" fracture, explodes bone and disc fragments into the spinal canal, sometimes with devastating results. Another fracture, a Chance fracture (first described in the mid-1940s by a doctor with the delightfully unlikely name of Quigley Chance), describes an injury in which the spine is literally pulled apart, at times right through the middle of the vertebra itself. As impressive as the X-rays appear, this type of fracture is seldom associated with nerve injury. Most patients recover fully after a relatively simple spinal operation and, occasionally, with no surgery at all.

### I have a friend who suffers from a segmental instability. What is it?

Segmental instability is another one of those terms that sounds worse than it actually is. "Segmental" refers to a motion segment, which is composed of two adjacent vertebrae, their intervening disc, and their linking facet joints. It is a useful biomechanical concept to understand spinal movement. "Instability" means that there is more movement between those two vertebrae than is considered normal. Unfortunately, experts can't agree on how much movement is normal, or whether that extra movement matters. We are not talking about a shift of a centimetre or two. Often the extra movement is measured in millimetres. To make it even more complicated, there is no uniform agreement among spine specialists as to whether or not that additional movement truly causes a failure of the linkage. Different clinicians have different definitions of segmental instability, and the only common factor appears to be that the term frightens patients.

### How do you define segmental instability?

I have borrowed a definition from a good friend of mine, an English orthopaedic surgeon, Steven Eisenstein. Steve describes what he calls ABC instability. The *A* stands for apparitional; in this case, the ghostly figure is on the X-ray. Many clinicians define segmental instability by measuring the difference in the position of the vertebrae on X-rays of the spine bending forward and X-rays of it bending backward. The *B* stands for biomechanical. Many studies in the lab have tried to establish the limits of normal movement. The *C* represents clinical. Many doctors and therapists use segmental instability to describe a pattern of back-dominant pain that is most intense when the patient attempts to straighten from a forward-bent position. When the normal spine straightens, it uncurls from the bottom up in smooth sequence. When a segment of the spine is deemed "unstable," there is a different and characteristic rhythm. The uncurling stops at the sore point, and a whole section of the spine seems to move as a bloc. The patients will often stop partway up, shift to one side, and resume straightening with a slight tilt. Sometimes they put their hands on their knees and push up.

It would be very helpful in understanding back pain if there were a correlation between apparitional, biomechanical, and clinical instability, but sadly, there is not. The only way we can reach any agreement is to first define the type of instability we are discussing. From a practical point of view, that makes the whole exercise frustrating.

There are a few instabilities about which we can all agree. One type is degenerative spondylolisthesis, where the worn facets allow the bones to slip. There is also the instability that follows major trauma, or the loss of large sections of the spine due to cancer. And instability can be produced by the surgeon who removes the linking joints during an operation. But for the most part, when the doctor talks about segmental instability, he or she is referring to the clinical sort. It is just another way of describing a back-dominant pain that comes on when you are bent forward. Sounds like Pattern 1 to me.

# CHAPTER EIGHT

## *Skydiving, Show Jumping, and Other Daily Activities*

After spine surgery, patients are always anxious to learn how soon they can resume their normal activities and what restrictions will apply. Usually, I impose very few limitations. My standard instruction is that they should avoid skydiving and show jumping for the first couple of weeks. Beyond that, they can do what they want.

I have similar conversations with the patients I see in the clinic who will never require an operation. It is only reasonable to wonder how the things you do every day affect your neck or back. All my advice is founded on the fact that necks and backs are not fragile and can safely withstand even the most strenuous daily routine. The information about carrying out the ordinary activities that make up our lives is generally simple and straightforward. Each pattern of pain requires additional specific recommendations.

**I spend my whole day sitting. Is that harder on my back than standing up?**

Sitting for a long time can give you a sore back. If you have Pattern 1 pain, it is important to maintain the arch in the small of your back with a large cushion or a twelve-centimetre (five-inch) lumbar roll. Patients with Pattern 2 may find that extreme position uncomfortable and are often better with a smaller roll or no extra support at all.

For both patterns, it is important to change position frequently. Pattern 1 patients should stand up, put their hands on their buttocks, and arch backward. Pattern 2s should stand up and touch their toes or just slump forward in the chair.

Most patients with neck pain will have Pattern 1, and they need to maintain the correct balance between their head and shoulders by practising regular neck retractions. Using a lumbar roll will encourage the correct neck-shoulder posture when sitting.

### When I am not sitting at work, I do a lot of bending. Is this a problem?

Bending forward can be very uncomfortable if you have Pattern 1 pain. The load on the discs, which are the most likely source for this pattern, increases as you flex forward. This pressure is even greater when you bend and then twist. Simply bending over to pick up something off the floor and then putting it to one side without straightening up or turning your feet can be a real grabber. Try to bend your knees. If you are moving things around, stand up before you turn. And move your feet so that your whole body turns, not just your back.

In complete contrast, Pattern 2s love to bend. Their idea of a good time is an hour or two crawling around the garden. Because their back pain is never worse with flexion, either during movement or as a position, bending is no problem.

Obviously, staying in any position for too long can cause discomfort for both Pattern 1 and Pattern 2. The strength and the endurance of the muscles along the spine becomes the limiting factor.

### I don't mind bending so much. It's the lifting that gives me trouble.

Lifting is a very complex activity, and there are many theories about the "correct" lift. As with so much in neck and back care, what feels best for you is probably your right way. Lifting requires strength. If you are not strong enough in your shoulders, back, and legs, the best techniques in the world will not prevent you from feeling pain. Unfortunately, the opposite is not equally true. Having the strength is no guarantee that you won't hurt.

The only undisputed principle of good lifting is that the closer the load is to your body, the less the load is on your spine. It's a simple question of levers. The weight of the object in your hands is multiplied by the distance of the object from your spine. Holding a weight straight out in front of you increases the load on your back by a factor equal to the length of your arm. Hugging the object is easy when it is a loved one or a baby. It is considerably less appealing when it is a bag of garbage or an engine part. But your back can't tell the difference and it doesn't care.

Much has been said about the importance of using your legs when you lift. The idea is that you transfer much of the work from your spine to the large leg muscles. That should give your back a rest. In practice, few people actually follow this advice. Studies show that it requires more energy to use your legs. Your body finds it more efficient to lift with your back. It shouldn't surprise you that your body will instinctively choose the easy way.

You may notice that if you are doing a lot of bending and lifting, the pattern of your movement changes over time. As your back muscles fatigue and the discomfort increases, you will automatically begin to use other muscles or other postures to help ease the strain. Kneeling down to pick up a load may not be your first choice at the start of the day but it may be your only option late in the afternoon. Unfortunately, using alternative bending techniques can increase the risk of back injury because they employ poor body mechanics and unusual muscle actions. Having sufficient muscle strength and improving your techniques go a long way toward solving the problem.

**What if the things I lift are too big and bulky for me to hold close?**
Awkward lifts always pose a problem. Most objects have a side or a corner that will give you the best possible approach. Take a moment to plan your lift before you start. When the load is large, using your leg muscles as well as your back makes a lot more sense. Consciously involve your legs in your plan.

At work or at home, help is often available if you take the time to ask. Doing something alone and doing it in a hurry is not always the quickest way when you factor in the time you spend in spasm or the fact that you will be unable to lift at all the next day.

In many situations, mechanical lifting aides are available. Something as simple as tipping a large box onto a dolly and rolling, rather than carrying it, may ward off your back pain.

**When you have the box on the dolly, is it better to push or pull?**
That depends partly on your pattern of pain. Pulling is easier and allows better control of your posture. For some Pattern 2s, pushing feels better because they tend to be more flexed.

**When I do a lot of lifting, my neck hurts. I am not lifting with my neck, so why do I get the pain?**
Lifting involves not only the muscles of your legs and low back, but the muscles in your arms and across the top of your shoulders as well. Jutting your head forward provides more leverage for the shoulder and upper back muscles and adds a little strength. When you watch people trying to lift heavy objects, you will notice that one of the first things they do is stick out their chin. Arching the neck and pulling the chin up tightens the small muscles at the base of the skull. Maintaining that tension can give you neck pain and headache. If you watch well-trained weightlifters, you will see how they deliberately keep their heads balanced above their shoulders.

**Is that also why they keep the barbell so close to their body?**
That reduces the load on the spine, of course. One of the most difficult lifts is to raise something over a barrier when you can't hold it close. Two classic examples are lifting a baby out of the crib and a heavy package out of the trunk of a car. The crib side or the lip of the trunk forces you to reach out. You must improvise to reduce the distance between you and the object. Coax your baby to the side of the crib. Put your foot up on the back bumper and lean over the trunk, or climb right in to lift the package over to the edge. With a little ingenuity, most difficult lifts can be made easier.

When you turn with a load, take your feet with you. It may seem faster to shift some boxes by lifting and twisting, but I can guarantee that you will last longer if you take small steps to change direction during each lift.

### Sometimes just standing in line for a long time gives me a backache. Is that normal?

Standing puts less load on the back than sitting down, but holding any position for too long generates enough pressure to make your back hurt. Standing with one foot up helps, and so does walking around. Anything you can do that distributes the pressure around the spine can delay the onset of pain.

### What about activities that continually jolt the spine? Jogging, for example?

Jogging brings many musculoskeletal and cardiovascular benefits. But it is not my activity of choice for a sore back or neck. As you run, the impact of your heels striking the ground is transmitted up through your legs and pelvis into your back and on to your neck. Although the joints at your knees, hips, and the junction of the pelvis and sacrum all act to reduce the effect, a lot of the force still reaches your spine. When my back is bothering me, I can feel every step.

When you walk, and especially when you run, you rotate your pelvis and twist your back. This is a normal movement, one that your body is designed to accept. But jogging produces an exaggerated torsion that can be hard on the spine. Incidentally, that twisting motion is also the reason that jogging and power-walking are good for your waistline. The constant activity of your trunk muscles firms them up and helps reduce your belt size.

### It sounds like jogging does a lot of good things. Is there some way you can protect your back?

Yes, there is. Much of the back's protection comes from the strength in the supporting muscles. Strengthening these muscles should be part of your jogging routine. I will discuss particular exercises for the abdominal, paraspinal, and trunk muscles in Chapter 15.

One obvious way to protect your back when running is to limit your distance. Jogging five or six kilometres (three to four miles) a day should be well within the limits your spine can endure. Choose a good shock-reducing surface. Running on pavement or asphalt will obviously create more impact than running on grass or a cinder track.

Choose your jogging shoes carefully. Try to find shoes that are well-cushioned with good treads and a broad heel to minimize the impact of the heel landing and reduce excessive rotation in your legs. A few of my patients have told me that using custom-fitted arch supports (orthotics) greatly reduces their back pain, but this result is not predictable so I do not routinely prescribe their use.

### What about other sports where you land heavily on your feet? Sports like basketball?

Many of the same principles apply. One of the differences is that in basket-ball, baseball, or soccer, you start and stop running throughout the game. But each of those sports, and others like them, adds another element to the equation. They all require you to move your back suddenly and in several different directions. Keeping your trunk muscles strong is obviously important, as is selecting the best available equipment, including footwear.

Squash has a reputation as a back killer. The nature of the game (at least the way I play it) requires you to repeatedly lurch forward and suddenly twist to one side. These are both movements to which the back objects strongly. But playing squash won't harm your back, and developing strength and endurance in your trunk muscles can reduce discomfort.

### So are there good and bad sports for your back?

I don't think of them that way, although some sports do have bad reputations. Use common sense. If you're an out-of-shape middle-aged man with a sore back, I think you should decline a serious game of football with a bunch of oversized college students. But it's a mistake, in my view, to avoid a friendly game of basketball or an afternoon of tennis just because you have a little back pain. It's a trade-off; if you enjoy the game, your pain may be a small price to pay.

Years ago, I was given a booklet sponsored by a drug company to be used for patient education. One quick read-through and I knew I would never use it. It was filled with silly advice, but the silliest of all was a list of "good" and "bad" sports. Never mind that what's "bad" for one back patient might make another feel good. This list played it so safe that it was laughable. I could imagine the company lawyer saying, "Look, we can't afford to have our name on this booklet if there is even the slightest possibility of somebody getting hurt after taking our advice."

The result was that virtually every popular sport appears in the "bad" list: tennis, golf, squash, basketball, volleyball – you name it. The "good" sports column was limited to such activities as non-competitive swimming and slow walking. I am surprised they didn't include tiddlywinks, window-shopping, and indoor bird-watching. The underlying message was that people with neck and back pain had to be so careful that they couldn't have any fun. That's nonsense.

### Obviously, you're not about to give me a list of good and bad sports.

Almost every sport puts some strain on your back, and virtually every back can stand it. If you are trying to decide which sport might work best for your back, divide the possibilities into three categories: those that place extra weight on your spine; those that require you to arch backward suddenly or repetitively; and those that require you to bend forward forcefully or frequently. In each category, you can create a subgroup of sports that require vigorous rotation.

A good example in the first category would be weightlifting. Less obvious inclusions might be horseback riding, dirt biking, hiking with a backpack, or scuba diving when you're out of the water. For the subgroup with rotation, you could add the shot put.

Your back will be arched and flexed at some time in nearly every recreational sport: basketball, tennis, badminton, volleyball, hockey, baseball, skiing, rowing, archery, handball, racquetball, and swimming. Most of these activities require rotation as well, and in some, like canoeing, rotation is constant and unavoidable.

Your choice of sport depends first and foremost on what you enjoy. If back comfort is a major concern, make sure the sport's movements complement your pattern of pain as much as possible. Run through your categories to get some idea of the ones that suit you. The best approach is to give them a try.

### I've watched Tiger Woods swing. Surely that amount of rotation can't be good for your back?

No one knows for sure, but many back specialists suspect you are correct. Certainly, many golfers develop back pain, and back problems are a constant concern to the professionals. But amateur golfers don't come close to reproducing Tiger's swing. Whether or not his swing injures the back is an academic question (or wishful thinking) for them. Every golfer, however, can adapt his or her game to minimize the stress on the back. The older style of golf swing that relied more on shoulder and arm strength than on the elastic recoil of the lower back is still around, and is useful for people with back problems. Use a cart for your clubs. When you finally get to take the ball out of the hole, use the golfer's lift; lean on your putter, rotate forward through one hip, and stick your other leg out behind. Your back hardly moves.

### What about sports like bowling or curling?

These activities would be included in that first category, exercises that place extra weight on your spine. Because of the position you assume, they also fit into the third group because they require you to bend forward. But the amount of weight isn't great, and the positions these sports demand would be ideal for someone with Pattern 2 back pain. Supplementing the sport with a few trunk-strengthening exercises would be a smart move.

### How is tennis on the back?

Squash may cause back pain, but I never understood why it took so much blame while tennis got off so lightly. A vigorous game of tennis requires you to arch your back forcefully then suddenly bend forward and twist. Except for the minimal weight loading (the weight of the racquet hardly counts), tennis puts your back through a real workout. If back pain is a problem, the game can be modified by changing your serve or taking up doubles.

### What about less organized sports, like hunting or fishing?
The less organized the sport is, the more freedom you have to make your own rules and find ways to be kind to your back. If you go fishing or hunting in the woods, pack light and let someone else portage the canoe or carry out the moose. Deep-sea fishing can pose a real challenge. Any contest with you and a big fish on opposite ends of a line for an hour or so will truly test your back. Try to position yourself in a balanced posture, use your arms and legs to share the strain, and get your trunk muscles in shape before you go.

### How about hockey?
Skating with your stick on the ice forces you to maintain a flexed posture for long periods of time. Add sudden twists and the occasional body check, and hockey becomes a great way to get a sore back. But like all sports, hurt is not harm. The fun of the game may more than compensate for the temporary discomfort it causes.

### So what about skydiving and show jumping?
Aside from the obvious risks, both are sports that load the spine. With a modern parachute, it is possible to land gently. A good horse rider takes most of the impact through the thighs. I always mention these two sports, not because they were particularly bad for the back, but because they are so far beyond most patients' everyday activities. It's my way of saying that almost any activity or sport is possible with back pain. There are virtually no limits if you do things the smart way. And besides, the notion of being skydivers and show jumpers makes my patients smile.

### What about less dramatic activities, like riding a bicycle or using a treadmill?
Exercise equipment allows for a controlled environment. The speed, resistance, and angle of the treadmill can be varied, and similar changes can be

made on an exercise bicycle. These adjustments allow you to modify your posture to accommodate your pattern of pain. Both Pattern 1 and Pattern 2 back-pain patients should be able to develop comfortable routines. You can avoid unwanted neck pain by keeping your head balanced over your shoulders to distribute the load evenly. Whether you run or bike inside or outside, the key is to not let your back pain stop you from enjoying the things you want to do.

Having back pain is not fun, but there can be a reasonable trade-off. Two of my patients serve as excellent examples. Neither is an exceptional athlete, though both enjoy their sport. One is a middle-aged man with Pattern 1 pain. He lives to play hockey. During a tournament, he may play two or three games over the weekend. His back pain can get so bad that he has difficulty bending forward to lace up his skates. Occasionally, it is severe enough that he elects to leave the game. But he knows that he is doing himself no harm, and he keeps coming back for more.

The other patient, also middle-aged, is an avid windsurfer. He has Pattern 2 back pain. I can't think of a sport where the back is arched more consistently. He has told me how much his back can hurt, but you would have to lock him up to keep him off that sailboard.

Both men put up with pain in order to participate in the sport they enjoy so much. I think that is a smart choice, and so do they.

### I don't mind hurting a bit if it's fun, but what if my job gives me back pain?

There are a lot of jobs like that, I agree. Earning a living isn't always as enjoyable as we'd like it to be. And some jobs do carry a higher risk of back problems. One of the most carefully studied risks is the effect of whole-body vibration. Truck and bus drivers and heavy-equipment operators are frequently subjected to this type of motion, and it has been shown that, at certain frequencies, the vibrations can actually accelerate the progression of wear within the spine. Of more immediate concern to the driver or operator is the fact that they suffer neck and back pain.

There has been much research into the best ways to dampen the vibration. Designers have developed seats that can cushion the effect. Despite a great deal of progress, the problem has not disappeared completely. But at least we are now aware that sustained exposure to vibration can be bad for the back.

## What other occupations are particularly difficult for people with back problems?

Except for vibration exposure, the connection between back and neck pain in any specific occupation is difficult to establish. We know that the incidence is higher in some jobs but we not sure if that represents cause or effect. Does heavy work cause back pain, or does back pain just interfere more with heavy work?

One way to aggravate back pain is to alternate between a sedentary activity and sudden heavy lifting. This happens, for example, with a truck driver who does his own loading and unloading. He works hard loading his truck for an hour or two, drives for several hours in a poor sitting posture, then jumps out of his cab and begins hoisting heavy crates again. It is the same story for bus drivers who must load the passengers' luggage under the bus, drive for a considerable distance, then unload the luggage when the bus arrives. Construction workers, dockhands, and nurses are all vulnerable because of the amount of bending, lifting, and twisting that they do. Claims for back and neck pain often include a report of either an unexpected lift or what I call the "slip and not fall." The first situation occurs when the future back-pain sufferer begins to lift with a co-worker and then the other person lets go. In the second scenario, the worker slips on a wet patch on the floor/ground and twists suddenly to avoid falling down. In both cases, the unexpected load catches the back muscles by surprise, and the spine has to take most of the strain.

A vintage example of a job associated with back pain is mining. Although machines now can carry out many of the hardest tasks, miners are still required to manoeuvre heavy vibrating equipment, shovel for hours, and carry heavy loads. The digging and lifting is often done in awkward positions and confined spaces that make good body mechanics impossible.

A jackhammer operator working on a paved street is slightly better off. The equipment is heavy and vibrates, but he can change his position and avoid twisting his back unnecessarily. More and more of this type of work is being replaced by sophisticated machines. Still, the connection between back pain and manual labour remains strong.

One thing that does matter is how much you enjoy your occupation. One study looked at truck and bus drivers. It examined the amount of vibration they experienced and how much they enjoyed their jobs. The truck drivers endured the most vibration and they had the highest degree of job satisfaction. They also had the least amount of back pain.

As we solve the problems in one area, other difficulties emerge. Ever-increasing levels of neck and back pain are being experienced by assembly-line workers, clerical workers, and especially workers such as call-centre operators who sit in front of a computer screen all day. The spine complains about heavy lifting, but it's not happy sitting still, either. The answer is to mix routines whenever possible. Find ways to reverse a frequently held posture or repeated movement. If you spend your time bent forward looking down, break the routine by arching backward and looking up. Don't wait until the pain starts. Do it before you get sore.

**So blue-collar and white-collar workers both experience back and neck pain. Does anyone escape?**
Not many. Firefighters face a particularly daunting challenge. It's hard to think of a way to place a greater demand on someone's spine than hurriedly climbing up and down a ladder under the most stressful conditions while toting a heavy fire hose or carrying a victim to safety. I have talked several times to a young man, the son of one of the nurses in my operating room, who cannot go back to work with his fire company because of his back pain. His symptoms are clearly Pattern 1. His pain is increased by any attempt to bend forward (as firemen do when they climb a ladder) or lift (as firemen do all the time). Not surprisingly, passive therapy and pills haven't worked. He is a strong and healthy young man with physical capabilities that already exceed those of most people, but for his back, in his job, it is not enough. It remains to be seen whether further intensive exercise to strengthen his trunk muscles will help. I hate to admit defeat, and I consider recommending a change of job because of back pain a failure. But you

can't win them all, and sometimes a strategic withdrawal may be the only reasonable choice.

Right up there on the list of things that are hard on the back is flying a helicopter. In flight, the pilot has both feet elevated to operate the rudder pedals. This sitting posture puts considerable extra load on the discs. Both arms are in use, so there is no opportunity to transfer upper body weight onto an armrest. The engine vibration never stops. I once treated a firefighter whose second job was as a helicopter flight instructor. I can't think of a worse combination.

### Those are some extreme examples. What about the things the rest of us do, like yard work?

Climbing a ladder to clean your eavestrough may be much less stressful than climbing into a burning building, but the position of your back will be the same. Shovelling a little topsoil may not compare to working on a construction site, but for a Pattern 1 pain sufferer, it will still hurt. So will raking leaves when you are bent forward and rotating all the time. Fortunately, working at home has one great advantage. You can pace yourself and stop if your back or neck pain gets too bad. The leaves will still be there tomorrow or, if you are lucky, they may have blown away (a technique my neighbour calls "passive yard maintenance"). Pacing yourself to get the job done without provoking the pain is an excellent strategy. This is especially true when it comes to shovelling snow.

### What is so special about snow shovelling?

It has been estimated that the cardiovascular effort of shovelling the driveway is similar to the same amount of time working in a mine. It's little wonder that every winter brings reports of heart attacks and back pain.

The first principle in snow shovelling is to pace yourself. If you don't get the job done all at once, the snow will wait for you to return, unless it melts in a sudden thaw (more passive yard maintenance). Dress warmly, particularly over your back. Cold air can tighten the muscles and make them sore.

When you shovel, lift light loads. Lots of small shovelfuls are better than fewer heavy ones. Carry the snow to the side rather than trying to hurl it a great distance. If you do throw the snow, turn your feet to face the direction you want the snow to go. Don't twist your spine and throw it to the side. There are specially designed shovels with curved handles that allow you to remain erect when the blade of the shovel is on the ground. If shovelling snow hurts your back, getting a back-friendly shovel may be a good investment. Whatever design you choose, keep the shovel light and don't fill it too much. Of course, there's always a snowblower, but wrestling one through a snowdrift may not be an improvement over smart shovelling. The flexed posture needed to drive a snowblower could be aggravating for a Pattern 1.

Similarly, cutting grass can be trouble for someone with Pattern 1 pain. A self-propelled mower may help, and a lighter electric model can ease the burden on your back. Find ways to change your posture. Plan your attack on the long grass. Work in stages, one section at a time. Alternate your grass cutting with other chores to give your neck and back a chance to change positions.

One activity I do not recommend you alternate grass-cutting with is hedge-trimming. Whether you do it with hand clippers or a power trimmer, the job demands a lot of time with your arms raised and the trimmers held at arms' length. This posture puts significant strain on your neck. If you are working on a low hedge, there is an added load on your low back.

If you are hauling firewood, carry small loads and introduce some variety. For example, you might carry the wood in a relay pattern: several trips from the wood pile to the bottom of the porch steps, then several trips up the steps and into the house. That way, the job becomes less of an endurance test.

The general approach to all these tasks is the same. Only the specifics are different.

### I guess the same applies to indoor chores?

Yes, it does. Vacuuming seems to be the one chore people complain about the most. Using the average vacuum cleaner requires you to bend forward over and over. The solution is to keep your back in a comfortable erect position and advance with your arms and legs. Try switching to the other hand; it's awkward initially, but you can acquire the necessary skill. Imagine handling it with the grace of a fencing master.

If you are making a bed, try to bend at your hips and keep your back relaxed or even slightly arched. You can bend at your knees if that doesn't take up too much energy, or you can tuck in the sheets and blankets while you are kneeling beside the bed. Try standing at the bottom of the bed and casting the sheet upward rather than pulling from the sides. And unless you are expecting a visit from royalty, learn to tolerate a few wrinkles here and there.

In the kitchen, keep a footstool handy. Straining to reach a high shelf is an invitation to aggravate your sore neck. Kneel down to reach into the lower cupboards and arrange the pots, pans, and heavy, awkward items in easy-to-reach places.

At the ironing board, try standing with one foot up on a footstool. If your back is really sore, try ironing while sitting down or perched on a high stool. Change positions frequently.

Standing to wash the dishes is another good time to use the footstool. Move around often. Give your back a rest once in a while by leaning your arms on the sink to take the weight off your upper body.

**I see what you mean about the basic principles being the same. Back and neck care doesn't sound very complex.**
It's not. A lot of it is just common sense. Because the advice is so simple and can be very repetitive, it's no wonder that patients who hear it in my office are often disappointed that I have nothing more elaborate to offer. But if it were actually as easy to live this way as it is to talk about it, then most of those people wouldn't need to see me at all.

It's easy to recommend regular exercise but it's hard to find the time to do it in the middle of a busy day. It doesn't require a lot of insight to realize that bending backward occasionally feels good when bending forward all the time hurts so much. But that doesn't automatically translate into action.

It always surprises me when people dismiss the obvious, simple solutions to their problems. It disappoints me when their lack of understanding and their fear of what might happen prevent them from taking control.

# CHAPTER NINE

## *Sex and Pregnancy*

**H**ave you ever considered that the time-honoured "Not tonight dear, I have a headache" may actually be a statement about poor cervical posture? A sore neck or a sore back can have a devastating effect on sexual function, and that loss of function can erode a relationship. In addition to the physical disincentive of back pain, both back pain and sexual activity have physical, emotional, and psychological factors that can complicate the situation. The emotional and psychological consequences of neck or back pain can be very powerful.

Back or neck pain can cause sexual failure; the failure causes negative emotions; negative emotions enhance the pain; more pain perpetuates sexual failure. Sexual inadequacy feeds on this loop. It causes enormous stress, and can be a source of anger and a prime reason for depression. All of these emotions will worsen the sufferer's experience of pain. But sexual disappointment is not a purely personal affair. An apparent lack of sexual interest in one partner may ignite a flare of anger and mistrust in the other. Both may become overwhelmed by frustration and a sense of hopelessness.

For many people, talking about sex in any form is difficult. Discussing sexual positions in detail can be downright embarrassing, but unless sexual problems are addressed openly and reviewed candidly, no resolution is possible. The pain-free partner often worries that the sexual rejection is not really due to a sore neck or a bad back, but is symptomatic of a deeper problem in the relationship.

And for the person with the pain, it may be less unsettling to dwell on the problem in your back or the trouble in your neck than to talk about problems with your relationship or trouble in your romance. But if your spine is destroying your sex life and you want to reclaim it, there are things that you and your partner can do.

### Rebuilding a sexual relationship is a terrifying challenge. Where do I start?

A loss of sexual ability does not have to mean a loss of sensuality. Feelings of love and romance can exist outside the sexual act. I am not minimizing the importance of sexual contact, but if your neck and back pain is hampering your ability to have intercourse, then it is probably not the place to begin.

Realize that your pain may have consequences that you both must bear. Start by openly discussing the problem. As gently as you can, explain why your sex life is not as good as it was. This should not be a clinical discussion. Plan an afternoon or an evening or, better yet, a weekend away in a location that is romantic or fun for you both. It's a good idea not to start in the bedroom. Pick somewhere new, with no reminders of previous problems. Try to ensure that you won't be interrupted. Be gentle, take it slow, and don't be afraid to cry.

### I don't suppose we begin by discussing the missionary position?

No, you don't. That will come in time, but first you need to re-establish a sense of intimacy and mutual trust. You both need to have confidence that each will consider the other's needs. Don't underestimate the devastation that back and neck pain can have on your relationship. What may have begun as one person's relatively simple physical problem can become a morass of emotions: fear of the pain, anger at the inadequacy, resentment, and guilt.

**I can understand that the partner with the sore back would be afraid. Where does the guilt come in?**

Sooner or later, both parties will feel guilty. The person with pain may feel remorse for failing in the relationship, for refusing to try to have sex. He or she may wonder if the pain is real, or if it's a subconscious way of avoiding intimacy. The partner may feel guilty about pursuing the idea of sex when it is obviously so unpleasant for their loved one. And there may be feelings of inadequacy, because what was once so wonderful has deteriorated to painful drudgery. Both may be resentful; one resents the pain, the other resents the unwillingness to try. At this stage, discussing these legitimate emotions and concerns is much more important than deciding on the best position.

**What if one person says quite honestly, "I can't have sex. It hurts too much"?**

In some cases, for a short while, that may be perfectly true. But often it needn't be. It becomes true because of the way people react to the pain. It is a self-fulfilling prophecy.

Picture it: two people go to bed, intending to have sex. One of them starts to groan softly, not with sexual arousal but because his back hurts. As the moaning grows louder, her attention shifts from his male anatomy to the anatomy of his spine.

"Is it your disc again, dear?"

"The pain is running right down my leg. I think I've pinched a nerve this time."

We will leave the scene before they begin to discuss the patterns of pain. But what chance do they have now of successful lovemaking? They might as well be sitting fully dressed in the clinic.

**Is their concern justified? Can intercourse harm your back?**

No, it can't. This is not an illness or a progressive, destructive disease of the spine. We are talking about mechanical neck and back pain, the patterns of pain that arise from physical problems in the discs and small joints. Intercourse, like any repetitive back movement, can cause pain, but it won't cause damage. Still, the fear of pain is genuine, and sometimes it is that fear more than anything else that stops couples from trying. But there is a world of difference between hurt and harm. There are things you do every day to all parts of your body that cause temporary pain but no permanent damage. Pinching your skin, stubbing your toe, biting your tongue, or having sex when your back is not at its best may hurt a little, but you won't be irrevocably injured.

But there are real risks to denying yourself and your partner the opportunity for intimacy, pleasure, and gratification. When I hear of people avoiding sex because of a bad back or a sore neck, I always suspect there is something else wrong with their relationship. Without either partner being aware of it, pain, or concern about causing pain for the other person, may have become the acceptable reason for saying no. It seems to me that if all other aspects of the relationship are in good shape, the appropriate response should be, "Let's try. Even if it hurts, it will sure be worth it."

## Do you often hear sexual complaints in a spine practice?

No. The subject is seldom raised by the patient, but the concern is there if I inquire about it. Many spine specialists are quick to focus on the mechanical or neurological elements of the back or neck problem, and never get around to asking whether there is any sexual dysfunction. For the doctor as well as the patient, it is a delicate issue.

Back examinations are seldom carried out in what you would consider a counselling environment. I see many of my patients in a clinic where conversations in one room could be overheard in another. Patients don't seem to mind much if someone hears them telling me about their back or neck pain, but they are not about to broach the subject of sex.

Even in the best of surroundings, it can be a difficult conversation to initiate. I remember a woman who came to me with back pain about six months after her marriage. Her husband came with her. After my examination, I was confident that her problem was simple Pattern 1 mechanical pain, and I started to provide her with the basic information for controlling the symptoms. At that point, she stopped me and whispered that she and her husband would like to speak to me somewhere where no one else could hear us. We found a quiet office away from the other patients and staff. As soon as the three of us were alone, I began to understand the real reason my patient had come to the clinic. She and her new husband had experienced an excellent sexual relationship before they were married, but now they were having serious problems. Her back pain was interfering with their sex life. She couldn't lie on her back and it hurt to put her legs in the right position. She got even more pain when she tried to raise her hips. She simply could not perform sexually; it was all too painful. She was really frightened that her marriage would fail because of it.

I have no way of knowing if her fears were well-founded. Usually, when I talk to a couple, I am repeatedly assured that the pain-free partner is understanding and willing to wait. I certainly hope that's true. But there are many times when a look or a comment has lead me to believe that the relationship is already in serious trouble. In those cases, the neck or back pain has acquired additional significance, and resolving the problem takes a lot more than a few sloppy push-ups, or a couple of retractions.

## Do men with back pain have the same sort of sexual problems as women?

Yes, they do. Back and neck pain makes vigorous performance in a man extremely difficult. And they have one other obvious problem: they can become impotent.

In most cases, this doesn't mean there is a serious problem. Most men with chronic back pain who fail to get an erection do so for more psychological than physical reasons. There are rare situations where impotence is due to reduced blood flow to the penis or damage to some of nerves in the pelvis, but these are extremely unusual and, for the most part, completely unrelated to the back pain. Impotence can be a problem in the older male population, where it is almost always associated with generalized blood-vessel disease. In the case of a younger man, whose failure to achieve an erection appears along with the signs of general disability from his back problem, it's not likely to be physical at all. Sexual dysfunction is one of the many hallmarks of pain-focused behaviour, and I will discuss it again in Chapter 10.

## So impotence with back pain is usually psychological?

Not quite. It may just be the pain. During an acute episode, sex may be so uncomfortable that the pain genuinely stops the action. Pain can be a sort of natural contraceptive.

But when a man remains impotent even when the back pain is not severe, there is a good chance that emotional factors are involved. He may fear that intercourse will bring on another attack of severe pain. The fear of sudden severe pain is almost as effective as the pain itself in inhibiting desire. And I can't think of a quicker way to lose an erection than to be stabbed in the spine by an excruciating spasm. Or he may be trapped by those unpleasant emotions in the cycle of pain causing sexual inadequacy, building frustration, leading to despair, accentuating the pain. And there's always the unhappy prospect that, back pain or not, he just doesn't find his partner sexually attractive any more.

## Do you think a man could just ignore the emotions?

He can certainly try, but it will not be easy. All these emotions are very powerful. In some cases, it might be easier to accept the pain and the limitations it creates than to admit the death of the relationship.

Failing to achieve an erection is almost invariably frightening for a man, and that fear can perpetuate the failure. The more he worries, the less likely he is to be successful. Achieving an erection occurs when your mind is focused on arousing images. It is not something you initiate by mentally reviewing potential vascular problems in your personal anatomy.

## What about medication?

The drug most frequently used for erectile dysfunction acts by relaxing certain muscles in the penis to promote easier inflow of blood and establish an erection. Its effect is produced by blocking specific local chemical reactions. But the series of reactions is triggered by sexual arousal. Without that first step, the drug has nothing to act upon. For a man whose impotence begins with back pain, it is the initial arousal that is lacking, and the action of the drug comes too late in the process to be of value.

**So a positive attitude is important to having sex with a bad back?**
Attitude is important and so are body mechanics. Once you and your partner have decided that having sex is a good idea, it comes down to technique.

**What is the best way to start?**
Sexual contact, with or without neck and back pain, should begin with foreplay. This includes a whole range of activities involving touching, gentle massage, oral sex, and other erotic behaviour. The encounter should be soft and tender, paying special attention to those things that make the spine feel better. An erotic neck massage can provide the best of both worlds. Prolong the foreplay as much as possible. The more you are aroused before actually engaging in intercourse, the less vigorous effort will be required. For partners who have avoided sex for some time, the foreplay may seem awkward. Don't try too much too fast. If it feels good, there will be a next time.

**When the time is right, how do you choose the best position?**
When you deal with back and neck pain, it is always a question of trying out the options. The partner with the sore back usually takes the more passive role in the lovemaking. He or she should find a position that supports the back or neck in a comfortable posture and should be required to move as little as possible. The pain-free partner should take the lead but keep the movements slow and easy.

**Do the patterns of pain help determine the positions?**
Yes, they do. But actual experience takes precedence over theory. You may select your original positions based on your pain pattern, but the ones you continue to use will be the ones that feel best.

Because people with Pattern 1 pain usually feel better with their back extended, they are generally more comfortable on top. The missionary position, with the lovers face-to-face, is the easiest way to start.

If the partner with back pain is experiencing a severe episode, he or she may be more comfortable underneath, regardless of the pattern. Both partners should help arrange this position with support under the low back and perhaps a pillow to elevate the buttocks. The knees should be bent to tilt the pelvis and take strain off the lower back.

### What if bending forward feels better?

If the woman has the back pain, she can kneel over the man and straddle him. Bending forward and keeping the weight on her arms will keep her back flexed. Although he is on the bottom and lying on his back, he is the pain-free partner, and should do most of the moving.

If the man feels better in a flexed position, the partners might try having intercourse while he is sitting up and she is sitting on his lap. Because he has the pain, she will need to be the one who moves, usually by bending and straightening her legs.

### That sounds a little too energetic for me. What positions produce the least stress on the back?

The spoon position can be very gentle. Both partners lie on their sides facing in the same direction. The woman is in front and slightly higher up the bed. The man lies behind facing her back. In this position he can enter her from behind. The depth of penetration is reduced and the action of intercourse can be very gentle with both partners contributing.

A variation is with the woman lying on her back while the man lies on his side facing her. He positions himself slightly below her and lies at an angle so that their upper bodies are apart. She now bends her legs up to allow him to come closer then drops her legs over his, keeping her knees bent. They are now in contact and he can enter her from this position. Once again, the act of intercourse is slow. In this position, only the man can provide the movement.

### From your descriptions, I can't be sure whether those positions would be more comfortable if you have Pattern 1 or Pattern 2.

And it doesn't matter. Whatever position works is the right one for you. In general, positions that promote back extension are better for Pattern 1. For the woman, this could mean lying on her stomach while the man enters her from behind. Her amount of extension can be adjusted by lying over extra pillows. The woman can also maintain back extension if she sits on his lap. We have already described that position as one that is comfortable for a man with Pattern 2 pain. With a little planning, even if both partners have pain, they can find a way to accommodate. Another position that promotes extension for the woman is kneeling on her hands and knees. She may position herself on the bed or kneel with her upper body on the seat of a chair or the side of the bed.

For the woman with Pattern 2 pain, flexing forward helps. We have already described positions where she can straddle her partner and then bend forward. Lying on the bottom in the missionary position works as well, as long as there is adequate support under the pelvis to maintain low back flexion. This position also maximizes penetration.

For the man with Pattern 1 pain, the missionary position usually works. However, completing his thrust puts his back into flexion. He should begin slowly, and gradually increase the range of movement. Just as the amount of back movement increases as you repeat your sloppy push-ups, the amount of back movement will increase as intercourse continues. It is the same principle of repetitive stretching. The man with Pattern 1 can also gain low back extension by lying on his back with a rolled pillow or towel for lumbar support. As his partner is on top and pain-free, she should be the one who moves.

Selecting the best position when you are a man with Pattern 2 pain can be tricky. He can, of course, just lie still in a comfortable position and let his partner do the work. But if he wants to take a more active role, he will need to find a way to avoid repetitive extension. If the woman supports her pelvis on several pillows she can lift herself high enough that the man can kneel with his knees below her buttocks. With her legs around his waist, he can enter her as he leans forward. Most of the rear-entry positions will also allow the man to have active intercourse in flexion.

### What about getting a book on sexual technique?
I think that is an excellent idea. It should give you a variety of ideas. Just exploring the possibilities with your partner can be foreplay. Whatever

keeps your back comfortable and does not embarrass you or your partner should work. Mind you, if you show up in the bedroom one night with an ironing board, a block and tackle, and a set of shoulder straps, you might not receive the response you were hoping for, no matter how good the position might make your back feel.

## What about sex after back surgery?

That will depend upon the type of spine surgery you have had. If the operation was only a small decompression, the only limiting factor will be the soreness in your back muscles. Sex should be possible as soon as you have the desire.

If you have had a larger operation, like a spinal fusion, there will be more pain, and your surgeon may caution you against vigorous movement during the first few weeks. But sex with a sore back is both possible and pleasurable as long as you choose the correct technique.

## Sexual activity can lead to pregnancy. For a woman, doesn't that mean more back pain?

Many women with back and neck pain are afraid to become pregnant because they believe their pain will get much worse, or they think that a bad back will prevent a normal delivery. Neither fear is justified.

It is certainly true that pregnant women have back pain, but the pain is generally temporary, intermittent, and creates no permanent problem. The patterns of pain are the same, although there is a higher incidence of Pattern 2 (pain with extension). Back pain in pregnancy begins most often around the fourth or fifth month. Although it can continue for the rest of the pregnancy, it often disappears for a few months, only to return with a vengeance during the final weeks.

There is no basis to the fear that mechanical back pain will interfere with normal delivery. Having a baby produces its own pains. Any previous back complaints will be quite secondary.

**Many women get an epidural injection for their labour pains. Can that cause back pain after the baby is born?**

This is a widely held belief and it is absolutely false. The epidural injection is a needle that delivers a short-acting anaesthetic inside the lower spinal canal but outside the sac containing the nerves. There are a few different routes the needle can take to reach its target, but regardless of the approach, it is only a single injection. Sometimes a small plastic catheter is passed through the needle and left within the canal for the duration of labour, so that additional anaesthetic can be administered as required. Once labour is over, the catheter is withdrawn.

Sticking a needle in your back cannot possibly damage the discs, joints, muscles, or ligaments that contribute to mechanical back pain. The needle track heals rapidly. The needle never passes through or even touches the principle pain sources.

Many women tell me that when they had the epidural injection, they felt a sudden pain in their leg. That may mean that the tip of the needle briefly entered the nerve sac and actually touched a nerve. Although that can cause a momentary flash of pain, a brush with the needle tip causes no damage. Even if it did, the symptoms would not be back pain. Nerve involvement causes leg-dominant pain.

**So why do so many women have back pain after the baby is born?**

Carrying a child for nine months places an enormous strain on a woman's body. There are massive hormonal changes that alter the amount of body fat, loosen ligaments, and stretch muscles. By the time the baby is born, most women have lost a significant amount of the muscular support around their midsection. The muscles of the abdomen are weak, the muscles across the floor of the pelvis have been stretched, and the muscles along the spine have lost their endurance. The weight of the pregnancy has added an extra load to the discs and small joints. Those discs and joints need more protection than ever from the physical stresses of everyday life, and there is no muscle strength to provide it.

As if all that was not enough, caring for a baby places new demands on the back. Lifting diapers and dirty laundry as well as the adorable newborn puts loads on the spine that often lead to mechanical pain. The patterns and pain-control strategies remain the same. Pregnancy won't change the nature of the problems, but it can intensify them.

### How can a pregnant woman control her back pain?

One small piece of good news is that you won't have to cope with the low back pain that many women feel during menstruation. That pain is the result of the hormonal shifts and fluid retention that accompany a normal cycle. But pregnancy replaces menstrual pain with a more mechanical one, and the mechanics begin to change early. Even before a pregnancy is obvious to the casual observer, most women show a characteristic gait that is quite different from their normal walk. The woman leans back a little, although the weight of the early pregnancy doesn't require her to do so, and her toes point outward. But for the disparaging overtones, I would describe it as a pregnancy waddle.

The changes in the way a woman walks are indications of the major changes that are beginning to take place in her body. The ligaments of the pelvis are loosening, so that when the time comes, the bones of the pelvis can separate enough to allow the baby to emerge. This altered structure changes the way her muscles act.

As the pregnancy progresses, the weight of the foetus and the increasing size of her abdomen force the pregnant woman to walk with an increasing arch in her low back, shifting her centre of gravity and changing the way she loads her spine.

Still, the patterns of pain are no different. Many pregnant women hurt more when they bend backward, but some have typical Pattern 1 pain. With a larger abdomen, the woman's range of movement is reduced, so a lot of the pain is postural rather than activity-related.

### So being pregnant is a guarantee of back pain?

Not necessarily. I have seen a few women whose typical mechanical back pain disappeared when they were pregnant. Pregnancy gave them the most lasting pain relief they had experienced. For most women, however, back pain is part of pregnancy. But it doesn't necessarily follow that suffering severe pain with one pregnancy will guarantee problems with the next. Because the pain is mechanical, and because it relates to the way the spine is loaded as well as to the amount of wear that is already present, the amount and location of the pain can vary. Although it is very uncommon, pregnant women can even rupture a disc and develop Pattern 3 pain from a pinched nerve.

### Are there any special rules for managing back pain in pregnancy?

Nothing more than you expect. Because of all the increased demands on her body, a pregnant woman needs adequate rest. When she lies down, she should support her spine and her pregnant abdomen. A pillow between the knees often helps. So does a lumbar roll. The changes in body mechanics can also cause neck pain, so proper neck support is useful.

Exercise is important. Prenatal programs generally include an exercise routine focusing on the muscles in the pelvic floor. Other exercises are designed to strengthen the abdomen. I recommend including exercises to strengthen the paraspinal muscles, the two ridges of muscle that run down the back. As you will see in Chapter 15, many back-strengthening exercises require you to lie on your stomach. A woman in the latter half of her pregnancy may find this impossible. There are alternative exercises that would be acceptable.

Modifying normal daily activities can also help alleviate back pain during pregnancy. Women with Pattern 1 pain who formerly found relief in high-heeled shoes will find this changes. Pregnancy increases the lumbar lordosis, and accentuating it further may be too much. Most women find flat shoes more comfortable.

The woman should ensure she is sitting properly. A lumbar support is helpful, and most pregnant women get additional comfort from using a small footstool. Standing with one foot up reduces the increased strain on the low back.

All of these things – rest, exercise, and changes in lifestyle – should be continued after the baby is born. Exercise is particularly important. Women often ask me how soon after delivery they can begin to work out again. Barring any complications of pregnancy, and with the consent of the attending doctor, I recommend they begin exercising as quickly as possible.

**So back and neck pain in pregnancy is just the same old back pain we have been talking about?**

Almost. There are two additional conditions that should be discussed.

The first is pain arising in the sacroiliac (SI) joints. These are a pair of large, virtually immobile joints that separate the base of the spine (the sacrum) from the large wings of the pelvis (the ileum). Part of the relaxation of the pelvis in preparation for delivery includes relaxation of the SI joints. That loosening can cause pain.

Sacroiliac pain produces a typical pattern distinct from the four patterns I have already described. The pain is located deep in the buttock, and although it occasionally radiates into the upper leg, it is clearly buttock-dominant. The pain is constant. It is different from the pain of a sore hip that increases briefly each time the hip takes weight on that side; SI pain continues and increases during the day, but it is more affected by general activity than by any specific movement. The one big exception is twisting in a chair or rolling over in bed. Both of these actions immediately produce the typical pain.

Like the patterns of back pain, the history of an SI complaint should be supported by the physical examination. I use several tests that are intended to reproduce SI pain. They consist of applying pressure to specific areas of the pelvis from the front, the side, and from behind. Here's one test you can try yourself. Lie on your back and place the foot of the painful side on top of the opposite knee. If you imagine the position of your legs, you will see why it is called the "Figure 4" test. Press your bent knee, the one on the sore side, down toward the floor. If this causes your familiar buttock pain, you probably have sacroiliac pain. Most people in that position will feel pain in the groin or tightness in the muscles of the leg, but that doesn't count.

**What can you do about sacroiliac pain?**

The pain is generally temporary and usually disappears when the pregnancy is over. For some women, it occurs during the middle months of the pregnancy as the SI joints loosen, then disappears before the baby is born. Besides the obvious measures of increasing your rest in comfortable positions and avoiding things that make the SI hurt, there are two things you can try. One is a sacral belt. There are commercially available belts that fasten snugly around the top of your pelvis. They aren't tight enough to actually stabilize the bones, but the pressure around the pelvic crest does reduce the pain. During one of her pregnancies, my wife used my broad, leather jeans belt to produce the same effect.

Sometimes SI pain responds to a stretching exercise that I call "knee to arm pit" rather than "knee to chest." Using your hands, draw your knee upward and pull it off to the side toward your shoulder rather than straight up onto your chest. The combined flexing and rotating movement may give some relief. Frequent sessions with five or ten repetitions each time seem to work best.

### You said there were two special circumstances with pregnancy. What is the second one?

I have already talked about a condition in the spine called spondylolisthesis, where one vertebra slides out of place over another. The disorder was first described in 1782 by a Belgian obstetrician, and for over two hundred years it has been recognized as a complication of delivery. When the spondylolisthesis is very pronounced, the bones of the spine actually slip so far forward that they lodge at the top of the pelvis in front of the sacrum. This abnormal position fills the upper birth canal and makes normal vaginal delivery impossible. When it was first identified, severe spondylolisthesis was an insoluble problem, and fatal for both the mother and child. Today, delivery can be accomplished successfully with a Caesarean section.

Having the vertebrae in the spine slip out of position is an unusual occurrence. Having them slip so much that they interfere with delivery is extremely rare. That degree of slip is easily recognized by the family doctor, spine surgeon, or obstetrician long before problems might arise. Once its presence is known, spondylolisthesis constitutes no real threat. Although it may occasionally determine how the baby will be born, it will not prevent a happy conclusion.

# CHAPTER TEN

## *Unfortunate Behaviour*

We are about to cross the boundary between what can be considered a straightforward mechanical problem and enter the world of pain-focused behaviour. It is a murky world indeed. Until quite recently, the model that doctors used to explain pain was over three hundred years old. First formulated by the French philosopher René Descartes, it assumed that pain was an accurate reflection in the brain of something that took place at the outer limits of the body. Doctors learned that particular types of nerve cells transmitted certain types of pain, and that these signals passed unchanged from the cut finger, the sprained ankle, or the bulging disc to the surface of the brain where they were recognized and recorded as pain.

Over the last half-century, and increasingly in the past decade, we have begun to understand the true nature of pain. Pain is not a report; it is a construct. The electrical impulses generated by a cut on the finger travel through the nerves of the arm and the nerves inside the spinal canal to enter the back of the spinal cord. From there, they progress upward into the brain, not as a single electrical signal but as a message passed from relay station to relay station. At each station the signal is either amplified or reduced until it reaches the conscious levels of the brain in a completely different form from the one in which it started. How much the finger hurts is determined not just by the severity of the cut but, more significantly, by how the information is transmitted. And that transmission can be amplified, diminished, or blocked altogether.

We know some signals coming from the body never make it to our consciousness. We routinely screen out much of the input that bombards our senses. Sitting at the movies, absorbed by the action on the screen, you are unaware of the texture of the seat, the smell of buttered popcorn, or the faint hum of the air conditioning. Some of these signals are dismissed by your brain; others never reach it at all.

Over the past thirty years, medicine has accepted a theory of nerve transmission that describes an electrochemical "gate" at the entrance to the spinal cord. This gate may be opened or closed by other stimuli or by signals sent down from the brain. An open gate means that the message from your cut finger enters the spinal cord and can proceed to the brain. But the gate can be closed by another signal that supersedes the pain of the cut. This is the basis of counterirritation. Rubbing on liniment that irritates the skin sends a message that closes the gate and reduces your awareness of the muscle pain beneath. The gate may also be shut by nerve centres within the brain itself. The wounded soldier who feels no pain until he notices blood on his uniform is the classic example. Presumably, his brain kept the gate closed during a life-threatening situation.

To make matters more complex, the system can also generate pain when none should exist. It has been known for generations that someone with an amputated limb can still feel pain in the missing hand or have an uncontrollable itch on the absent foot.

Researchers are discovering more and more about the transmission of pain within the spinal cord and the brain itself. It is a complex chemical and electrical process that is mediated by a large number of enzymes and other chemicals. It can be adapted and shaped. There are even visible structural changes inside the brain and spinal cord that develop in response to a prolonged exposure to pain.

One thing is absolutely clear: the pain is real. Some of us do hurt more than others, and that hurt is genuine. The pain, controlled by the gates and modulated by centres in the brain, may have little resemblance in character, duration, or intensity to the original problem: the cut or the bulging disc.

Our state of knowledge is, in many ways, comparable to the situation medicine faced with tuberculosis one hundred and fifty years ago or, more recently, with the HIV virus that causes AIDS. We recognized the pathogen (the infecting agent) and we understood the process by which it ravaged the body, but we could not make it stop. There was no cure and very little control.

Chronic pain can be equally overwhelming. Although we understand its mechanisms and its progress, we do not possess the direct means to make it stop. We do not have a drug, a device, a treatment, or an operation that can abolish this type of pain. When the pain we feel is a reasonable representation of the problem in the periphery, treatment at the site will work. Removing the irritating pressure of a bulging disc on an exiting nerve will cure Pattern 3 sciatica. But when the pain resides in the central nervous system and is disconnected from its original source, we have no way to touch it. It remains beyond our reach, where it can take over and destroy a normal life.

### I've had back pain for years and years. Do I have chronic pain?

In one sense, you certainly do. The word chronic can be used to indicate simply that someone's back or neck pain has been present for a long time and is well past the acute-onset stage we covered in Chapter 5. But that is not the type of problem I am talking about now. We're dealing with a more complicated and, in almost all respects, a more serious problem. I am talking about your emotional and psychological reaction to long-lasting pain. I am talking about behaviour. People who come to focus on their pain change the way they act. Pain becomes the centre of their life, and every decision they make is based upon how much they hurt.

Several years ago, I was moving into a new house and I needed light fixtures. I found a small store that seemed to have everything I wanted, and on my first visit I made several purchases. The clerk, a middle-aged man, was quite attentive and helpful. When I paid, he noticed that my credit card had "Dr." stamped on it and asked me what kind of doctor I was. I told him that I was a back doctor. The floodgates opened. My sales clerk had chronic spine pain and had already undergone two surgeries on his neck and three on his low back, none of which was completely successful. Because I had been paying attention to my lights, I had not noticed the small wires running from the inconspicuous electrical stimulator in his shirt pocket over his collar to the pads on his neck and back. He went on and on with far more enthusiasm than he had shown in selling me the fixtures.

I made frequent visits to the shop and each time, my special clerk sought me out to update me on his latest crisis or triumph. On his good days, he was helpful and would bring my purchases right to the counter. On bad days, when his pain was severe, he couldn't lift even the lightest box, so I took to going into the stockroom to get the items for myself. He was very apologetic, but his pain would not let him help.

When I had all the lights I needed, I stopped going to the store and lost contact with the clerk. Some months later I went back for an additional item, and found that he was no longer employed. The manager told me that he had been forced to let my clerk go. His good days and bad days made him quite unreliable, and he had annoyed several customers with his lengthy descriptions of his pain.

This man had obvious pain-focused behaviour. He did not fit the common but inaccurate stereotype of the chronic pain patient: the bedridden, housebound female. He was a man who was attempting to work but whose pain had become such a focus in his life he could not escape.

### That sort of behaviour seems very self-destructive.
It is certainly very unfortunate. Focusing on pain will actually increase the severity, and that is the last thing that you want. The pain focus will also drive people to seek short-term relief, and this makes them easy prey for anyone who promises to help. These are the patients who fill the clinics offering a quick fix through massage or electrical therapy. These are the patients who seek out the doctors offering local-anaesthetic injections.

And these are the people who keep going back to the chiropractor or manual therapist. In the end, pain takes control of their lives.

### Is their pain imaginary?

The term doctors use for pain that arises from an emotional or mental conflict is "psychogenic pain." It is a poor description because it leaves the impression that the pain is not real. Nothing could be further from the truth. These unfortunate people really do hurt more.

### Where does the pain come from?

The pain develops within the central nervous system itself. A number of changes take place within the spinal cord and the nerve centres in the lower part of the brain. Through chemical and structural alterations, patients develop a central sensitization and experience pain when there is no reason for them to. It is as if they become aware of the normally insensible workings of the nervous system, and all these routine, regulating mechanisms become painful.

### That sounds awful, and I can see it is a real problem. What is the best name to describe it?

We don't really have one. Many names have been tried. "Myofascial pain syndrome" is one. In English, that just means the pain seems to come from the muscles and fibrous tissue of the body. "Regional pain syndrome" is another attempt. As the name suggests, it indicates that the pain is not related to a specific structure but tends to spread through entire areas of the body. "Chronic pain syndrome" is the term that I used for many years. A syndrome is a collection of signs and symptoms for a condition without known cause. So we are talking about a definite pattern associated with chronic pain. It's a good description, but the term has begun to have very negative overtones. It can also be easily confused with any pain of long duration. Currently, the terms that are used most often are pain-focused, illness, or disability behaviour. Although each has a slightly different implication, they all refer to the same problem. The terminology changes, but the condition doesn't.

## Aren't they just malingering?

Malingering means "to pretend to be ill or otherwise incapacitated in order to escape duty or work." People who exhibit chronic pain behaviour are not pretending. Their behaviour is erratic and pain-centred, but they are consistently that way. Pain-focused patients have good days and bad days, like my sales clerk, but they follow their own cycle, not one that is scheduled to deceive. Malingerers put on a show when it is required, for instance, when they appear before the Pension Review Board. The rest of the time they can and do behave normally. Although malingering is talked about a lot, it is actually quite rare.

Of course, patients with pain-focused behaviour sometimes exaggerate their symptoms as well. That is only natural. It is a characteristic we all share. The exaggeration will depend upon the circumstances. A medical assessment, particularly when there is an evaluation for financial compensation involved, is a good reason to make your symptoms obvious.

A family physician told me an engaging story. One of his patients, accompanied by her ten-year-old son, came to his office seeking a medical certificate for total disability. The doctor questioned her about the seriousness of the problem.

"It's awful," she groaned. "All I do is cry."

"I've never seen you cry," her son said.

"I cry all the time," countered the mother. "My pain is so bad I can't even do the laundry."

"I've seen you doing laundry," piped up the little boy.

The doctor told me his patient got no support for her disability. He was not sure what her son got.

Lest we get too judgmental, remember that all of us behave in that same way. Circumstances often dictate how we react to pain. Imagine you have just won ten million dollars in a lottery. You are on your way with the winning ticket to the lottery office when you slip and twist your ankle. I guarantee that in your enthusiasm to get the money, you will hardly feel the pain and you won't limp at all. Now imagine you are on your way to the dentist for root-canal work. You have been dreading the visit for weeks, and on your way out of the house, you slip and twist your ankle. The pain is excruciating, and certainly bad enough that you must postpone your appointment.

We should not forget that patients suffering pain-focused behaviour are in many ways no different from us. They respond to their circumstances, just as we do. They just hurt more.

### I am confused. Is this type of chronic pain a physical problem, or is it abnormal behaviour?

It is both. There is a genuine physical basis for the problem in the altered anatomy and abnormal chemical reactions within the brain and spinal cord. Although we understand these changes, we cannot yet do much about them directly. The increased pain of the central sensitization affects behaviour and, for now, the behaviour is the only thing we can treat.

### How can treating behaviour solve the pain problem?

I admit it is a very indirect method, but at the moment, it is the best we have. Everyone, including the patient with a strong pain focus, will agree that pain affects behaviour. You act in a way that supports your pain. In my whimsical moments, I see the pain as a malevolent creature looking somewhat like a large, brown gopher living inside the victim's body. Whatever the gopher wants, he gets, by pushing the right button or pulling the right string. Every time pain makes you do what it wants, the pain gopher wins and you lose.

But it is a two-way street. Not only does pain affect behaviour, but behaviour can drive away pain. Every time you act as if there is no pain, in other words, every time you act normally, you and not the pain gopher push the button or pull the string. It means that you are in charge and you regain control of your life. The theory is that modifying behaviour sends a message to the sensitized central nervous system that somehow resets the mechanism. That input seems to do what medicine can't yet do; return the pain-reporting process to normal.

**That doesn't sound easy.**
It definitely is not. And before I can even begin to discuss strategies for the management of pain-focused behaviour, I have to be sure that a pain focus, not an obscure mechanical cause or underlying illness, is the source of the patient's problem.

**How do you do that?**
The first steps are taking the patient's history, performing the physical examination, and ordering any necessary special tests. If I identify a simple mechanical pattern in the midst of a pain-focus problem, I deal with the mechanics first.

People who develop this serious behavioural illness tell a story that is remarkably consistent. So consistent, in fact, that it is usually possible to be certain of the problem just from listening to their history.

The story often starts with two proud announcements. The first is that they have a very high pain tolerance. The second is that all they want to do is get better and go back to work.

Unfortunately, pain tolerance is like gas in the tank of your car. The further you go, the more you use until you run dry. Patients with chronic pain have had a great deal of experience with pain but they have long since lost their tolerance. They just don't realize it.

A colleague of mine who runs a pain clinic sometimes asks a group of patients to line up along one wall of the room and then arrange themselves according to who feels the most pain – the worst in one corner and the rest in descending order. Invariably, this request creates a small stampede. Everybody in the class tries to get into the corner reserved for those with the worst pain.

When patients say that they want to get better and go back to work, it may be the truth, but it also hides a number of problems. In most cases, patients with pain-focused behaviour have come to see themselves as victims and have transferred control of their lives to someone or some-thing else, usually that cursed gopher with the buttons and strings. They do want to get better, but they are not willing to take the responsibility or do what must be done. Their wish to return to work is not as clear-cut as it sounds, either. In many cases, people with chronic pain have left jobs they didn't enjoy in the first place and to which they never want to return. Wanting to go back to work really means wanting to return to a job they have never actually had, for which they are not qualified, which will not worsen their pain, and which is better than the one they held.

## Are there any other characteristics of pain-focused behaviour?

There are many identifying features. Here they are in alphabetical order.

### Assistance with Personal Care

These people see themselves as too sick to do almost anything. Here is an excerpt from an actual disability review:

> ... his wife attends to his daily needs, washing and dressing him as well as shaving him and brushing his teeth.

It is hard to conceive of any mechanical pattern in either the neck or low back that would require such a level of personal care. But it is not unusual in people with pain-focused behaviour.

### Blaming Others

Being a victim is a big part of pain-focused behaviour. It doesn't start that way, but as the sufferer's life disintegrates, it becomes increasingly necessary to find someone to blame. Without an external villain, the sufferer will be forced to look inward, and that is the last place he or she wants to go.

### Constant Pain

Because pain is a constant focus, the pain itself becomes constant. People with pain-focused behaviour will have good and bad days, days where they can do almost everything and days when they can do nothing at all. But although the pain may relent, it never disappears completely.

Constant pain can be part of Pattern 1 and Pattern 3. It may indicate underlying disease or non-mechanical spinal problems. Taken by itself, constant pain tells you very little; when it is combined with the other components of pain-focused behaviour, the connection is obvious.

### Demanding a Physical Diagnosis
No one with pain-focused behaviour will easily admit that the problem lies in his or her behaviour. Everybody resists the idea that their pain is emotional or, even worse, an indication that they are not coping well. They must have a physical reason for their plight and that reason is usually related to the site where the pain first began. Obtaining an authoritative structural diagnosis becomes one of their major ambitions.

### Expanding Array of Symptoms
Mechanical neck and back pain stay in one place. At most, the natural process of wear and tear will slowly spread to adjacent segments of the spine. Because patients with pain-focused behaviour are experiencing pain from a central location rather than a specific peripheral site, the pain may appear anywhere, and it does. What may have begun as neck pain after a rear-end collision will, over time, spread not only to the head, arms, and shoulders, but to the knees and ankles as well. There is simply no way that a purely physical problem can migrate around the body like that.

### Financial Compensation
I have already talked about the effect that the external environment will have on a patient's perception of pain. It is not difficult to understand that if the pain, pain that is genuinely felt, is the basis for financial compensation, then that pain will remain severe. It would be almost impossible not to be consumed by the symptoms and their impact on lifestyle. Adding a financial reward inevitably increases the pain focus. And it doesn't take very much. One study showed that when the average compensation award amounted to only 55 per cent of the pre-injury net income, the number of claims increased drastically.

## High Level of Previous Activity

One recurring feature of the history in pain-focused patients is how extremely active they were prior to the onset of the pain. I remember seeing one man who weighed well over 160 kilograms (350 pounds) who assured me that, before his accident four months earlier, he had been a world-class field hockey player. That may have been his perception, but I doubt it was the truth.

I do not believe that these people are deliberately telling me lies. But their perception of reality has been badly skewed. All of us tend to exaggerate our past physical exploits. Everyone who played sports in high school remembers being the star of the team. For patients whose lives have been eroded by pain, an activity as simple as buying groceries is elevated to an Olympic-level event, and they remember it that way. Relative to what they can do now, they may be right.

## Litigation

In the same way that financial compensation heightens the pain focus, litigation keeps the pain front-and-centre. If pain is the reason you hired a lawyer, and if the lawyer's job is to present you in the most tragic light, then the pain must be accentuated and displayed. For someone already dominated by pain, whose gopher has grown to an enormous size and controls all the buttons, adding a lawsuit cements the behaviour. The longer the legal confrontation continues, the stronger its effect. And it would be naive to suggest that there are no incentives for the professionals to prolong the process. If a case is settled quickly and inexpensively, there are no substantial legal fees. And there are fewer charges for conducting medical examinations and writing depositions. Many delays are unavoidable, but extending litigation has significant financial benefits for the law firm or medical practice.

In some instances, a doctor may unwittingly slow the process for fear of legal reprisals. If he or she is wrong in predicting the recovery outcome, the lawyer may sue the physician. So the doctor hesitates. "I can't be sure yet. I'd better see you again in six months." That means nobody is going to settle for at least that long, and the patient must sustain the pain. Medically, there is no basis for the delay. Without the threat of litigation, no competent doctor would wait six months before deciding on a course of treatment or giving the patient some idea of what to expect.

The course of litigation enhances pain-focused behaviour. Lawyers instruct their clients to maintain a "pain diary," a daily log of how much they hurt. A visible record of success is one of the elements of a good treatment routine, but a pain journal that has the patient review repeatedly how poorly they feel is a sure means of supporting the behaviour.

I once examined a mother, father, and three children, who were all involved in a lawsuit over a rear-end collision. No one had been seriously hurt physically, but the ensuing legal battle had a devastating effect on all of them. The suit became a family business. No one was going to let the family down by getting better. And no one did. They just kept on reinforcing each other's pain-focused behaviour.

Much has been written about the effect of a successful legal settlement on the presence of illness behaviour. Many doctors believe that once the lawsuit is over, the pain will disappear. Others are convinced that settlement will have no effect. I think the answer is somewhere in the middle. For a few claimants, whose situation was the major factor sustaining their pain, a successful settlement may end the cycle. For most people, the pain focus has become integrated into their personality, and no victory in court will salvage the disabled persona they have acquired.

One patient's comment was, sadly, all too typical. On the preceding visit, she had told me that her pain was gradually subsiding. Then the next time I saw her she said, "I'd almost forgotten about my neck pain but my lawyer told me to come back and see you to be reassessed. And so I started thinking about my pain again, and it came back."

## Multiple Consultations

For pain-focused patients, the search for a physical diagnosis never stops. When one doctor, therapist, or chiropractor admits defeat, it is time to move on to another. Unfortunately, many doctors are more than happy to assist in the search by ordering repeated tests and X-rays. Like the additional investigations, every added consultation brings new vindication and proof of the serious physical nature of the pain. The fact that no significant physical problem is ever found only confirms what the patient knew all along: the diagnosis is unusually difficult and a cure will defy medical science. Every time a physician or chiropractor agrees to search for a physical source, they validate the patient's concerns and thereby reinforce the patient's pain-focused behaviour. A bad situation is made worse by specialists who quickly criticize their predecessors, implying that only now has the sufferer come to someone who really knows what's going on.

Because of the negative impact of multiple consultations, I have sometimes declined to see a patient. I remember a man whose only contact with me was a letter he wrote from another city to ask whether I would diagnose the back pain that had troubled him constantly for twelve and a half years. The duration of pain alone ruled out virtually all the potentially serious causes. But there was more, significantly more. With his letter he enclosed a loose-leaf binder containing a neatly typewritten, fifty-five-page monograph entitled "A Patient's Perspective of His Own Back Pain." It came complete with appendices and a short bibliography. He had become so obsessed with his back pain that it had become his career.

## Negative Work/Family/Social Settings

Pain-focused behaviour is not happy behaviour. The victims are usually depressed, often hostile, and are totally accepting of their permanent, complete disability. They have become "professional victims" who think and talk about little else. It is a new vocation, and a demanding one at that. Their behaviour puts the people around them in a difficult situation. Do you accept the sufferer's disability and make allowances, help with chores, and offer all the support you can? Or do you try "tough love" and demand that the victim go it alone? Either way you lose. Giving in validates the behaviour. Withdrawing support will cause the pain to intensify and the behaviour will become more florid in an attempt to regain your attention.

## Poor Response To Medication

Since most analgesic medication is intended to treat peripheral pain, it has little effect on the pain of a sensitized central nervous system. But most pain-focused patients take it in large quantities. It is an obvious indicator that they are ill and have a serious problem. It is affirmation that the pain is severe, physical, and real.

The conversation always intrigues me.

"You're taking a lot of pain medication."

"I have a lot of pain."

"Do the pills help?"

"No, they don't do anything at all."

"But you are taking a lot of pain medication."

"I have a lot of pain."

"Do the pills help?"

"No, they don't do anything at all."

"But you are taking a lot of medication. . . ."

## Sexual Dysfunction

Pain affects performance. When that pain is part of a larger abnormal behaviour pattern, it may be impossible to resolve the sexual dysfunction component. And sexual failure, particularly impotence in a man, compounds the predicament. It typically directs attention away from the pain-focused behaviour as the cause, and toward a search for a non-existent physical explanation for the failure to achieve an erection. It becomes the perfect diagnosis for the patient who "knows" that a serious physical illness is the problem, despite a growing list of normal investigations. The sexual dysfunction is set apart from the abnormal behaviour pattern and becomes proof of the seriousness and obscurity of the problem.

## Sleep Disturbance

Any pain can disturb sleep, but pain-focused behaviour disrupts a normal sleep pattern over 98 per cent of the time. The areas in the base of the brain that process pain are adjacent to those that create anxiety and control sleep. There is a physical connection between a focus on pain and a failure to sleep.

Patients with mechanical neck and back pain may have problems sleeping because they cannot find a comfortable position. But that pain is local and predictable, and a solution lies in posture correction and physical manoeuvres for pain control. In contrast, the patient with pain-focused behaviour reports "never" sleeping. One woman told me that it had been thirty days since she closed her eyes. That is physiologically impossible. A complete lack of sleep causes psychosis and total collapse within a few days. But she was adamant that it was true.

The real story is nearly as devastating. Patients with pain-focused behaviour do not sleep normally and occasionally do not sleep at all during the night. They do fall asleep for brief periods during the day, but these intervals of non-restorative sleep are only enough to keep them alive, and far too little to let them function normally. Sleep deprivation itself can cause pain. Patients get locked in another cycle where pain interrupts sleep and lack of sleep causes pain.

## Unemployed

Like the clerk in the lighting store, few people with well-established pain-focused behaviour can maintain steady employment. Their ability to work depends upon the severity of their problem. Not all pain-focused patients are disabled. Symptoms range from a preoccupation with their pain, a trait that promotes frequent medical interactions, to a complete obsession, making normal relationships and work schedules impossible. Unemployment is more common in this group and, taken with the other typical characteristics, one more indicator of the loss of function that accompanies a focus on pain.

## Unexplained Deterioration

The pain of central sensitization fails to improve the way you would expect with a recent physical injury. Mechanical pain is aggravated by specific movement or position. It runs a predictable course that may be long but is finite. The pain that accompanies pain-focused behaviour is unpredictable and fluctuates for no apparent reason. Like sexual dysfunction, unexplained deterioration often raises concerns in the mind of the doctor. "Why isn't my patient getting better? What have I missed?"

Those misplaced worries can lead to another round of investigations and consultations, further validating the patient's concerns and strengthening their abnormal pattern of behaviour. What is actually being missed is the array of symptoms of a severe pain focus.

**That's quite a list. Are all the features important?**
Individually, none of them indicates illness behaviour. Taken together, however, they form an irrefutable body of evidence. In fact, if five particular characteristics are present, the probability of the patient having pain-focused behaviour is greater than 99 per cent. The five characteristics are:

- blaming others;
- financial compensation;
- litigation;
- negative work/family/social setting; and
- sleep disturbance.

**If pain-focused patients receive compensation for their pain, won't that encourage them to keep hurting?**
Yes, it can. That brings up the concept of secondary gain. The term describes any situation where someone with an injury profits from that injury by receiving benefits that would not have been available had the accident never happened. It is another demonstration of the fact that we each tend to respond to our situation. Obtaining secondary gain is not necessarily a bad thing, but it certainly reinforces a focus on pain.

The elements of secondary gain can be listed as an acronym: FACE.

*F* stands for financial. If someone's income depends upon their pain, they are obliged to keep hurting. And the pain is real.

*A* stands for affection. People with back and neck pain are frequent visitors to the doctor, chiropractor, or physiotherapist, where they receive care and attention that may not have been available in their pre-injury environment. Having someone who is concerned about you is a comforting thing. If receiving that concern depends on having pain, then the pain will continue. And if more pain means more concern, the pain will grow.

*C* stands for control. Having back and neck pain is an effective way to get people to do what you want, as in, "I'd love to help take out the garbage/do the dishes/wash the windows, but I have a bad back." Giving up the pain means taking on those jobs again. That may not be an appealing prospect.

*E* is for escape. Sometimes a sore neck or a sore back may be the only way out of a bad situation. I have been an orthopaedic consultant to many professional dancers. I have seen performers whose careers were faltering for lack of talent develop vague back or neck pain. Now they could say, "My career is through because my spine let me down." Their egos remained protected.

In a less dramatic fashion, the same escape can occur in any workplace. A worker's relationship with his or her supervisor and level of job satisfaction are better predictors of an attack of disabling pain than are the physical demands of the job. Many people have no choice but to earn a living at a job they dislike. When neck and back pain provide an opportunity to escape, the offer is too tempting to refuse. Once you start down that road, there is no easy way to turn around. Giving up the pain means going back to the very place you don't want to be. But living with the pain is a terrible price to pay. And as the effects of central sensitization advance, there may be nothing you can do to make it stop. Your new job as a professional pain patient will turn out to be worse than the situation you left.

## What about the physical examination?

Examining the neck or back usually shows a loss of normal movement and muscle strength. Chronic pain produces prolonged inactivity. Prolonged inactivity causes joints to stiffen. Stiff joints restrict movement, and the associated muscles become weak through lack of use. Trying to use weak muscles causes pain. And so, in the end, chronic pain reproduces itself.

In addition to the obvious stiffness and loss of strength, there are a number of other physical findings that doctors recognize. They are called the Waddell signs, named after the Scottish orthopaedic surgeon who classified them. These tests are a series of manoeuvres and movements that patients anticipate will produce pain but which do not. A pained reaction when none should occur is taken as an indicator that the patient is not reporting his or her physical condition accurately. It's easy to assume that positive Waddell signs mean the patient is lying. In fact, patients may truly be experiencing pain as a result of their central sensitization. It is not relevant that the pain has no physical basis in the back or neck. Because interpretation is so difficult, the Waddell signs must be used with care and, like the separate elements of the history, the physical test results cannot be taken as independent evidence of illness behaviour.

### Is this the same as fibromyalgia?

Fibromyalgia and chronic fatigue syndrome are closely related to the problem of pain-focused behaviour. Many people, and I am one, believe that they are simply different manifestations of the same problem. The current research into fibromyalgia is focusing on brain chemistry and neural transmission of pain, the same area under investigation for chronic pain.

My strong objection is not to the diagnosis of fibromyalgia; it is to the negative connotations and support system that have grown up around it. As far as I can tell, the system doesn't support the patient as much as it supports the disorder. Patients diagnosed with fibromyalgia are told that they have an incurable illness. They are introduced to a fibromyalgia clinic, where they attend regularly for an indefinite period of time to review their symptoms, receive medication, and take short-term pain therapy. It is so hopeless and so self-defeating. The label fibromyalgia allows the patient to continue as a victim, the victim of a disease for which we have no cure and from which there is no hope of recovery. I cannot think of a worse starting point to restore normal function.

I once interviewed a woman with fibromyalgia as part of a continuing medical-education program for family doctors. Her story contained most of the identifying features of pain-focused behaviour, and added the multiple tender points that are the hallmark of the condition. The woman was originally diagnosed by her husband who, while working as an appliance repairman, had a customer with fibromyalgia whose complaints were the same as his wife's. Once he had labelled his spouse, he began learning about the disease. He quit his job and started working for a local support group. He was in the audience at the educational session and quickly joined me at the podium to tell the audience of family physicians the "truth" about fibromyalgia. And, of course, his principal teaching aid was his wife. What hope did this lady have of recognizing her pattern of pain-focused behaviour as the cause of her troubles and taking back control of her life?

### What about treatment? With so many things going wrong, where do you start?

You start with the fact that the "pain affects behaviour/behaviour affects pain" equation works in both directions. You treat the behaviour, because you can't get to the pain. Short-term modalities or manual therapy may produce brief periods of comfort, but the pain will be back. Those short respites from pain can re-emphasize its return and these sorts of approaches can therefore actually make things worse.

My objection to pain clinics for treating pain-focused behaviour stems from the fact that even the name puts the focus back on the very thing that we should be trying to eliminate. Asking a pain patient, "How is your pain today?" is an invitation to review all the aspects of the problem. That is the wrong strategy.

Because changing pain-focused behaviour is so difficult, the first step must be to win the patient's confidence. Unless you can convince the patient that you really do care and want to help, the patient will have no trust in the difficult and painful program that must be followed. Telling them to get over it invites them to increase the pain behaviour to prove that it's not possible. Only when the practitioner and the patient are in agreement that something should be done can they move to the next step.

Pain-focused patients may be difficult to live or work with but they can be a pleasure to treat, just as long as you don't go beyond short-term pain control. They thrive on the secondary gain of affection. One patient I saw is the perfect example. He is a man we all called Norm, after the character in the old *Cheers* TV show. Norm was a patient in one of our CBI clinics for nearly nine months. He was off work and, so long as he was in treatment, he was receiving full benefits. Norm wasn't getting better, but that didn't seem to matter to him. He was unfailingly pleasant and cheerful. He brought the staff flowers and candy. He had learned and remembered everyone's birthday or anniversary.

I was in the clinic one day to see some patients when I saw Norm for the first time. As he walked through the front door of the clinic, he waved and everyone waved back. Everyone knew his name. We had a short conversation and I examined him. It was obvious that Norm was a patient with a well-established and completely accepted pattern of invalid behaviour. And he was charming. The only problem was that Norm was not working. The insurance company that paid for his time off the job was, understandably, increasingly reluctant to do so.

When I had finished my assessment and determined that Norm was physically capable of going back to work, I went out to the front desk and told the administrator that it was time for Norm to move on.

"You can't discharge Norm." She said. "The place won't be the same without him."

There is the problem. Patients with pain-focused behaviour develop an environment that supports their pain. It is, after all, their primary focus, and they work hard to ensure that it is everyone else's main concern as well.

### How do you break a cycle like that?

Sometimes you don't. The approach we have to take is lengthy and indirect. Technically, it's called behavioural modification and cognitive conditioning. Its basic assumption is that the patients' behaviour is determined by how they perceive their pain and how they interpret their situation.

Education is directed at providing a plausible explanation for the pain and its unusual characteristics. A basic knowledge of central sensitization is appropriate. The patient learns that the pain is real and also that the pain can be controlled, and permanent disability is not inevitable.

The program is designed to shift the patient's focus away from pain and onto something that he or she can change. The best place to start is with the daily schedule. Because these patients sleep poorly and are usually unemployed, they lose their regular routine. They sleep when they can, do a few chores on the good days, and hurt all of the time. Pain, not the clock, determines when they get up, when they lie down, and everything they do in between. To put pain-focused patients back in control of their lives, you start by putting them in control of their schedules.

## How do you do that?

I recommend that patients start a day planner: a notebook they can use to schedule their life beginning the very next day. With the help of their family, friends, or therapist, they plan each day, breaking it up into hour-long, thirty-minute, or even fifteen-minute blocks. They decide today what they are going to do tomorrow. In each time block, they put a little square to be marked off once they have done what was planned.

No matter how much they hurt at the time, they try to follow the schedule with no exceptions and no accommodations for the pain. If they are successful, they check off the box and move on to the next time period. If they manage to meet all the day's plans, they have a full set of positive checks and a visual record of their success. That tally is important. It is tangible proof that they, and not the pain, ruled the day. When the day's schedule is complete, they start planning again. And so it goes.

Success is essential, so the goals must be achievable. A reasonable starting point would be to schedule a walk, or to stand or sit for a period about half as long as it usually takes to produce the pain. Most patients worry about scheduling too much, but it can be just as much of a problem if they schedule too little. The patient sets the schedule but, once set, it can take no account of pain. It doesn't just enforce activity if the pain is severe; it may demand rest even when the pain is trivial. If the schedule requires an hour in bed, that must be adhered to even if it is a "good" day and the patient is anxious to be doing something else. It is the *schedule* that determines the events of the day, not the *pain*. That is a strange way to do things and it takes some getting used to.

## But don't most pain-focused patients try to be active anyway? That clerk in the lighting store did.

Yes, they do. Or at least, that is often what they tell me. They are quick to point out that even with their pain they have been able to walk, or sit, or stand, or whatever. Then they go on to discuss how much those things hurt and how proud they are of themselves for sometimes doing them in spite of the pain. Do you see the difference? Here, the pain is still in control. The patients' activities depend on whether it's a good day or a bad day. Their level of function swings as erratically as the seismograph tracing of an earthquake. In contrast, the schedule disconnects how much they do from how much they hurt. It's not the type or amount of activity that matters, it's choosing to do it with no regard for the pain. And the behaviour must be normal. That means no grimacing, no silent tears, and no moans of pain. It means no non-verbal messages to your friends and loved ones that you are being brave and carrying on in spite of it all. Normal people don't act that way.

Adhering to the schedule will flatten out the peaks and valleys. Days become more predictable and events can be planned without the usual "If my pain lets me, I'd love to . . ." The emphasis shifts from how much they hurt to how far they can walk, how long they can sit, how much they can lift, or how many times they can bend. These are all activities that can be objectively measured and recorded. Reviewing this permanent record is a crucial part of the positive reinforcement that pain-focused patients require to conquer their abnormal behaviour.

### Do they have to schedule everything?

Everything they can. It is particularly important that they schedule their sleep cycle, beginning with the time they get up in the morning. They can make their own choice – it is their schedule, after all – but once the choice is made, they must stick with it. It almost inevitably requires family support, but it needs to be done. The second part of sleep repair is to establish a bedtime and a bedtime ritual.

### How does a ritual help?

Any caregiver of young children learns that bedtime works best if there is a sequence of events culminating in the big moment. There may be a snack, a bath, brushing the teeth, pyjamas, then a bedtime story, good-night hugs, and, finally, lights-out. The precise routine doesn't matter, but having the routine does. The pain-focused patient who has lost his or her ability to sleep properly during the night needs to re-establish a similarly predictable ritual. There are a few don'ts for the time leading up to bed. Don't drink, don't smoke, don't eat a heavy meal, and don't exercise strenuously. Don't read or watch television in bed; that sends the wrong message. If you want to read or watch TV, do it sitting on a chair, and preferably in another room. The bedroom and the bed are for sleep and, if you are making real progress, for sex, but for nothing else. Good sleep is a habit that has been broken and needs to be restored.

## What else should be scheduled?

The other important issue has to do with medication. Most patients with pain-focused behaviour take large numbers of pills that don't seem to do very much good. Telling them to stop doesn't work. But shifting the same dose of medication to a timed distribution makes a lot of sense. When pain-focused patients take ineffective medication in response to pain, the pain decides the timing. Moving to a time-based approach is one more way of shifting the control away from the pain. Instead of the pain gopher telling the patient when to pop a pill, the pill will be popped when the patient's schedule says so. The total daily dose remains the same, but the schedule dictates when it will be available. Over time, and with the doctor's agreement, the amount of medication can gradually be reduced. The interesting thing is that the pain often falls into line with the schedule, and time-regulated medication provides better pain control, and at lower dosages.

## How long does all this take?

How long is a piece of string? I have seen some patients make progress within the first month while others struggle on for two or three months before giving up. As time passes, the schedule should become more ambitious and less detailed. It's not the writing in the book that matters; it's creating the attitude that says, "Every day, I will be in control." The written record is the proof. If there are gains in the amount of activity, then setting the schedule can be moved from a daily event to a once-a-week affair. That is an individual decision.

You need to map out the goals carefully. They must be measurable. Those little tick marks mean a lot. The goals must be achievable. Patients with pain-focused behaviour already see themselves as victims and as failures. Adding more failure makes things worse. And the goals must be directed by the patient. Having a doctor or therapist plan the schedule just means that the professionals are in charge instead of the pain gopher. That is not the answer either.

## Do some people regain control?

Yes, they do, but not often enough. Still, every once in a while, pain-focused patients can turn their behaviour around, and they are some of the most grateful patients I see. I remember one man who waited in my clinic for nearly three hours just to thank me for what I had done. Of course, he was the one who had taken charge and made it happen. My role had been to lay out the program, much as I have given it to you here, and then coach him along as he tried to change his behaviour.

Pain focus can develop at any age. I saw a seventeen-year-old girl who had developed illness behaviour after she broke her leg in a figure-skating accident. The fracture had healed, but the pain behaviour continued. I remember her well, not only because of her age, but because one of her scheduling dilemmas was how much time she should allot for hanging out at the mall. She did conquer her pain focus, a victory her mother termed "a miracle."

Most patients with fully established pain-focused behaviour are unable to stop all their pain medication. And that is not necessarily a bad thing. Following an unsuccessful spinal operation that left him with significant low back pain, one of my patients went on to develop most of the characteristics of pain-focused behaviour, including regular use of a large amount of narcotic painkillers. For two years after the surgery, we both struggled with his pain. Another operation was not possible, but his level of function was unacceptable. Gradually, he began to take charge of his problem, and little by little, he regained control of his life. The remnant of his pain behaviour now consisted of requiring one session of physiotherapy for hot packs and massage every two weeks, and taking a single dose of narcotic every night at bedtime. Within six months he had returned to work as a bailiff in a courtroom.

That return to work took place nearly twenty years ago. Since then I have seen this patient every six months to renew his prescription for the narcotics and to authorize his continued physiotherapy. I doubt the therapy serves any useful physical purpose, and I have certainly had to repeatedly defend extending his narcotic prescription. But his goal and mine was that he stay at work: and he did. John retired last year at age sixty-five. He retired with a perfect work record, having never missed a single day on the job in the twenty years since he returned. He was a man who had overcome his illness behaviour, and I was more than happy to support his two remaining concessions to his battle against pain.

I hate to be pessimistic, but the odds of overcoming a well-established pattern of pain-focused behaviour are probably no better than one in five. You certainly don't win them all, but it's always worth a try. I had a lengthy conversation with a twenty-one-year-old woman who came to me following a motor-vehicle accident she had been in nearly a year earlier. At the time of the accident, she had been attending school and hoping to get into law enforcement. Since the accident, she had received countless physiotherapy treatments providing passive therapy and short-term pain control. She had dropped out of school and had not bothered to check on the availability of future classes. She and her boyfriend were no longer physically intimate and, although she assured me that the relationship was not in trouble, I had serious doubts. Pain that had begun in her neck had now spread to include most of her body and, of course, she was sleeping poorly. Her lawyer was dealing with the insurance company regarding the amount of compensation she should receive.

I spent a long time talking to her about her problem. I outlined most of the points covered here. She was grateful I had been willing to give her so much time. And she was equally happy to return to her therapist to resume her three-times-a-week massage and hot-pack program. As we parted, she again thanked me for my encouragement and asked whether another CT scan might help locate the "real" source of her pain.

One of the difficulties about telling real stories about my patients is that you can't manage the endings. After I had finished writing the previous account, but before it was published, the young lady came to see me again. She came with a little notebook containing three months of her daily schedule and a big smile on her face. In her case, my pessimism had been unfounded. The pain-focused behaviour had evaporated. I was talking with a new person. Her account was a summary of the elements that mark success in overcoming pain behaviour. The original consultation had convinced her that her pain was real and not in her head, as all the other doctors had told her. She wasn't crazy. With that understanding came a plan, a map that could lead her away from her focus on pain. She and her boyfriend, now her fiancé, decided to take the journey together. If she forgot to plan her next day, he reminded her. Sometimes they worked it out together. She found a job and made a point of walking to work. Every day she made a plan, and every day she followed it. She contacted the school and enrolled in a new course. The most exciting part of her story was what she told me about her pain. Within of month of letting the schedule, not her symptoms, control her day, the pain started to subside. Most days now, she had no pain at all, and when it did occasionally appear, after she had been on her feet a long time, it was in one particular point in her low back. It seemed very strange to her that the pain was so local and predictable, and no longer roamed at will all over her body. She could identify a clear mechanical pattern. For the first time in a year, her body had resumed accurate reports of a minor physical problem. I may not be able to write the endings I want, but if that were possible, I couldn't have come up with a better one.

### If they can follow the schedule, do the patients just get better?

Not in a predictable fashion. Only one thing is certain. Every pain-focused patient who increases his or her activity will reach the point psychologists call "behavioural incongruity." In plain language, it means they reach a time when they realize that if they truly hurt as much as they believe they do, they can't possibly be doing all the things they are doing. At this crucial juncture, they have only two choices. Most often they will decide that the pain really is more than they can bear, and their rehabilitation fails. Less often, about 20 per cent of the time, they will decide that the pain isn't all that bad and, now that they are in control, they want to stay there.

I remember one woman who was working out at a CBI facility. I had business in the clinic on a regular basis and so I saw her in the gym week after week. I cannot recall a more unhappy person. She was going through the motions and was staying with it, but it obviously wasn't fun.

One afternoon, as I entered the clinic I passed a very attractive woman hurrying the other way. We almost collided and, as I stepped aside, she gave me a big smile and said, "And you don't even know who I am."

It was the woman from the gym. She had had her moment of behavioural incongruity just a few days earlier, and decided it was time to get on with her life. That image of the difference control can make will always stay with me.

My advice is not always well-accepted. I remember one woman I had advised to stop seeing doctors (including myself), to avoid passive treatments that offered only temporary relief, and to begin a regular exercise program. She ignored that advice and went on to see two other physicians. One prescribed massage. The other, an acupuncturist, stuck needles into her. Because both practitioners had offered to take charge of her problem while allowing her to passively await the results, she liked their treatments much better than my advice. But she came back to see me to say, "Well, your last bit of advice was no help. What are you going to do for me now?" I felt as though she had dealt me into a hand of poker and was challenging me to up the ante.

# CHAPTER ELEVEN

## *Call in a Specialist*

At some point, most people with long-standing neck or back pain will choose to see a specialist. And what a vast choice they have. Because back pain is so common, and because it has so many different aspects, there is a wide assortment of professionals willing to accept the mantle of expert.

The average family doctor makes no such claims, but still sees the majority of patients with spinal pain. A few studies suggest that a significant proportion of neck- and back-pain sufferers seek their first consultation with the local pharmacist. Then there are the exercise-class instructors, the fitness gurus, and even the health teacher in high school. Because back and neck pain are so common, virtually everyone has either had personal experience or been close to someone who has. All this familiarity generates a sense that everyone is an authority. Certainly everyone has something to say. I have long maintained that if you are travelling in a strange city and wish to strike up a conversation, the best way is to tell someone you have a bad back. Before long, you will be the centre of a small crowd of vocal advocates for one or another form of treatment.

When it comes to public perception, the chiropractor is an easy winner. A survey published in the United States in 2001 found that 61 per cent of patients believed a chiropractor's services are superior to conventional medical care for the treatment of neck conditions. Only 6.4 per cent believed doctors know best. For low back care, chiropractors were chosen by 46.1 per cent of the respondents. Only 12.4 per cent chose doctors. It is a similar story for headaches, with chiropractors receiving 39.1 per cent of the vote while doctors garnered only 19 per cent.

Why are chiropractors so highly regarded? There are several reasons. First, they address the patient's immediate concerns of pain control and reassurance far better than the traditional medical approach. Second, chiropractors generally employ manipulation, and manipulation often works. It was one of the treatments for acute low back pain recommended by the Agency for Health Care Policy and Research. Third, the average chiropractor is an excellent salesperson. You might consider that an unattractive attribute, but think for a moment of your approach to buying a car, a house, or a major appliance. One of the things that makes you feel most comfortable about spending your money is your confidence in the knowledge and integrity of the salesperson. Health-care delivery is no different.

Both commerce and health care demand an informed consumer. With so many options available, what you receive may be predetermined by the practitioner you chose. If you go into a hat store wanting to buy a screwdriver, you are more likely to come out with a hat than a screwdriver. The same limitations of options apply if you seek a surgical opinion from a rheumatologist, a physician who deals with the medical aspects of spinal diseases, or if you request a spinal adjustment from a neurologist, a doctor who, except for hitting one with his reflex hammer, has probably not touched a patient in years. A reporter for the *Wall Street Journal* took her aching back to eight different specialists and got eight different diagnoses. She saw an acupuncturist, a chiropractor, a homeopath, an osteopath, a physiatrist, a psychiatrist, and a neurologist. She even consulted a celebrity doctor. The cost of her visits ranged from $70 to $800, and no specialist completely agreed with any other.

Seeking an expert is not as straightforward as you would like it to be. Having some idea about their particular areas of interest will help. So will knowing the type of treatment they are likely to provide. Today, many patients come to see me with a large amount of information obtained from the Internet. They present me with the treatment options they prefer, whether I am in the business of providing that type of spine care or not. To reduce the frustration for both you and your chosen expert, it is helpful to know roughly what is in store. If you are certain that you don't want spine surgery and nothing will change your mind, why see a spine surgeon? I had a conversation with a patient like that. In fact, he came back three times to tell me he didn't want surgery. Then he announced he was going to see a neurosurgeon. I asked him why, since he wouldn't consider an operation? He was going to see what the neurosurgeon had to say.

Although spine-care experts are numerous, there is a limit to their availability. I make this point to try to gently discourage patients who come to me seeking their seventh or seventeenth opinion. I know that patients with pain-focused behaviour will continue to search for the real cause of their pain. I am referring here to the patient with straightforward mechanical pain who is simply not satisfied with what he or she has already heard. It may be reasonable to seek a surgical consultation if the medical one was unhelpful. I won't object if you would like a chiropractic assessment after your doctor appeared confused by your problem. But I draw the line on rendering the fourth or fifth surgical opinion. I remember very well one woman who brought her husband to see me. He had severe spinal stenosis, a narrowing of the spinal canal, and was suffering from incapacitating Pattern 4 leg pain. Quite correctly, the first three surgeons had recommended an operation to enlarge the space available for the nerves in his low back. The first opinion had been given over eighteen months earlier. I think the patient would have accepted an operation on the very day he saw the first surgeon. But for one reason or another, his wife was not satisfied, and so, over the next year and a half, she arranged for him to see two more spine surgeons, and then finally brought him to my clinic. All our opinions were exactly the same, and all of us offered surgery as the appropriate solution.

My office hasn't received a request to book this man's operation. I suspect his wife has moved on to another surgeon, pushing her husband along in a wheelchair.

### Where do I start? How do I pick the right specialist?

It helps if you have some idea of the nature of your problem. A medical diagnosis of an underlying illness or systemic condition will certainly change the type of specialist you should see. Your family doctor is often a good place to start. He or she may not be an expert in neck or back pain, but your own physician is in the best position to assess your general medical condition and to review your past medical history. If the problem appears merely mechanical, then your own physician is well placed to make the correct referral.

If you decide to seek help on your own, and if you are certain your problem is one of ordinary neck and back pain of the sort we are discussing here, then I recommend that you begin with someone who is easily accessible, relatively inexpensive, and who offers a primarily mechanical approach to the problem.

Your choice within any particular group will reflect your personal preferences. I suggest you look for someone to whom you can talk easily and whose explanations of your problem make sense. I would avoid someone who promises too much or who insists that you will require a lengthy, complicated course of treatment.

Mechanical spine pain should respond rapidly and a program of pain control should be completed within a few days or a few weeks.

My personal preference would be for a practitioner who helps me develop my own strategies for control, and who acts more as a coach than a health-care provider.

### Can a chiropractor do that?

Many doctors, especially family physicians, feel frustrated treating neck and back problems. The chiropractor has obviously received special training, and seems confident about handling the situation. Some family doctors establish a relationship with a chiropractor early in their practice and begin to refer cases. In the best circumstances, the referral works both ways. The chiropractor sends on people that he or she finds to have a medical problem.

### Are chiropractors medically trained?
Chiropractic has come a long way since the first chiropractic adjustment was given by D. D. Palmer in 1895. Chiropractic is based on the assumption that most of the body's ills arise as a result of structural problems within the spinal column. Adjusting the column to restore its health is the basis of classic chiropractic care.

Today, chiropractors are required to have a minimum of three years' undergraduate university training, then to complete a four-year course at a chiropractic college. Their studies concentrate on spinal anatomy and manipulation, but cover a wide range of other medical topics. There is a stronger emphasis on business management than there is in the average medical curriculum. At the end of their program, successful students emerge with a Doctor of Chiropractic (DC) degree.

### Is seeing a chiropractor a good idea?
Chiropractors are expert at providing mechanical hands-on therapy. Manipulation of the spine can be an effective way of eliminating acute mechanical pain. Its value and low level of risk are covered in Chapters 5 and 6. It is a reasonable option for many patients, and the chiropractor is a suitable provider.

My problem with chiropractic is not with the profession as a whole, or with many of its proponents. Chiropractic crosses the line when it begins to promote treatment for conditions that manipulation cannot address.

I recall being on a panel with a teacher from a large American chiropractic college. We were in front of a medical audience. He was asked whether spinal manipulation could treat diabetes. Diabetics suffer from a lack of insulin, a chemical produced by cells within the pancreas to regulate blood-sugar levels. There is no known connection between the function of the pancreas and the peripheral nerves that leave the spine in that area, although many chiropractors claim that adjusting the spine will have a beneficial effect on the disease.

The instructor chose his words carefully. He stated that it was clear that chiropractic adjustment could not treat diabetes. I was impressed. He went on to say that it was nevertheless wise to have the patient's blood sugar checked after an adjustment, since the manoeuvre could change the level significantly. In other words, the chiropractor can't treat diabetes, but he can adjust the body's blood-sugar levels. Masterful piece of double-talk.

For many years, chiropractors asserted that spinal manipulation could treat asthma. When they were attacked on the logic of that assumption (since there is no recognized connection between the peripheral nerves and the function of the small tubes in the lungs), critics were told that the proof of the statement would come from the results of an ongoing study assessing the value of spinal manipulation in asthma patients. Because the results were pending, no further proof was offered. Chiropractors continued to provide asthma therapy. The results were finally announced in the *New England Journal of Medicine* and they showed that spinal adjustment had no effect on the frequency or severity of asthmatic attacks.

Most chiropractors quietly dropped the treatment from their list of available therapies, although some still insist an adjustment has value.

I realize that chiropractors are not the only ones who base their practice on scant evidence or general consensus. A lot of doctors do exactly the same thing. Evidence-based medicine is a growing trend, and although it is far from universally accepted by physicians, it is even farther from the norm in chiropractic care.

### I heard a chiropractor say he could treat ear infections in children. Is this possible?

That has been a common claim for some time. It turns out that most ear infections in children recover spontaneously and no treatment is required. Spinal adjustment will have no effect, but at least it is not as harmful as the unnecessary prescription of antibiotics, which can create drug-resistant organisms and foster more dangerous problems.

The list of chiropractic claims is long, and includes straightening crossed eyes, improving your children's learning abilities, and retarding the ageing process. None of these claims is substantiated, and a large number of chiropractors are as frustrated as I am that this type of promise is still being made by some of their colleagues.

This raises another question, the use of spinal adjustment in children. One group of chiropractors has gone so far as to say that the process of normal birth damages the spine, and that every newborn requires early adjustment to grow normally. It always strikes me as odd that nature, after millennia of evolution, has arrived at a mammalian birth method that is inherently damaging to every newborn. Recommending you bring your baby for an adjustment may be a good way to enlarge a chiropractic practice, but it does nothing for the baby's spine.

### Is there anything wrong with manipulating a child's back?

If the adjustment is done carefully and gently, it will cause no physical harm. But it will produce no benefit, either. And developing a habit of regular chiropractic treatment has never been shown to possess the merit of regular visits to your dentist. Spinal manipulation in children cannot promote normal growth or strengthen the spine. It can create a sense of dependency and a belief that without the chiropractor's intervention, your back will never be normal.

### Why are chiropractors so popular?

For many reasons. First, their primary treatment tool, spinal adjustment or manipulation, does work well for acute neck and back pain. But there is much more than that. Chiropractors have mastered the art of building patient loyalty. Many are viewed as a family friend in the same way that the old-time, small-town family doctor was. Today, medical practices can be impersonal, and are frequently very busy. That personal touch has been lost. Specialists usually treat patients only once or for a limited period of time. If the treatment is successful, they may not see the patient again. That is no way to build a relationship.

A past president of the American Chiropractic Association once told me that chiropractors were kept busy treating patients with neck and back pain partly because doctors had relinquished the responsibility. He said, and I agree, that many MDs were not keen to treat spinal pain and were happy to let somebody else take it over.

Many doctors lack the ability to sound confident about most back problems. Imagine you are trying to decide between two investment brokers. Broker A. tells you, "I suppose we might, uh, find some suitable stock or bond for you, but the market is, uh, rather uncertain these days. Of course, I would be happy to look into it and do whatever I can, but I must warn you that I can't guarantee . . ."

Broker B. tells you: "Look, I've made a lot of people wealthy in the past five years. Seven of my clients had to borrow bus fare to get here. Today they are millionaires. I can do the same for you. This is my plan . . ."

As it turns out, broker A. is a far shrewder investor than broker B., but that will never come through during your visits. Salesmanship is not a dirty word, and I wish more doctors dealing with spinal pain sounded less tentative.

Then there is the unworkable medical model: the need to make an unnecessary diagnosis, or at least provide a list of frightening possibilities.

"Doctor, can't you make my pain stop?"

"Not until I make a diagnosis."

"How long will that take?"

"Well, it's hard to be specific until we run a few tests. We have to make sure it's not something serious like cancer."

Not exactly a reassuring exchange.

Chiropractors rarely fall into that trap. Chiropractic diagnosis is based on whether or not a manipulation will be effective. If manipulation helps, the problem is a "manipulatable lesion" (there's a mouthful). If not, the problem is "something else." That long list of frightening possibilities never shows up.

Chiropractors do tell many of their patients that their back has a curve in it and that one leg is a little longer than the other. All backs possess normal curves, and most of us do have a slight difference in leg length.

Neither fact is important, and neither contributes to simple mechanical back or neck pain, but patients don't know that. It's reassuring to them that their practitioner has found something that can be treated.

### But when I go to the chiropractor with my sore neck, I come out feeling better.

That is why so many people chose the chiropractor over the doctor for the treatment of mechanical spine pain. In many cases, I think that is a good choice. My concern is not with the use of adjustment. It is not a worry about safety. My concerns centre on the patient's need for self-reliance and the delivery of an erroneous message that backs are fragile and need to be tended by someone else. My frustration comes from watching people spend money for treatments that they believe will have a lasting effect. I would rather have them spend money to sign their child up for a soccer camp with lots of activity than pay the chiropractor for the child's adjustment. Manipulation works when there is pain to work on. It does nothing for the pain-free spine, and it is completely useless in preventing future attacks.

### But don't children get back pain?

Yes, they do. New research suggests they get it in remarkably large numbers. Up to one-third of adolescents complain of intermittent mechanical neck and back pain. But this pain is almost never the result of a serious problem. It is temporary and disappears by itself. Not surprisingly, it occurs most often in children who adopt the same poor spinal habits as their parents: avoiding physical activity, sitting in soft chairs, and watching too much television, for example. Back pain seems to run in families. It is more common in the children of parents who have had spine surgery. Whether it is genetic, the result of the family's lifestyle, or just imitation, is unknown.

Much has been said lately about the use of backpacks for carrying schoolbooks. Several researchers have looked at the weight of the pack and how it is balanced on the children's shoulders. Some of the statistics are quite surprising. Relative to their body weight, some students carry significant loads. Distributing the weight and balancing the pack are good ideas. Having your back adjusted doesn't address the problem. There is no correlation between backpack use and problems in the spine. There is an increased risk of injury, but it comes from falling off a bike or down the stairs because the pack is too heavy.

Most spine pain in children is best treated with exercise and lifestyle improvement.

### Can't the chiropractor prescribe that as well?

Yes, they can. Many do. More and more chiropractors are recognizing the importance of including regular exercise and lifestyle prescriptions in their treatment plans. So are many doctors. Although we are still a long way apart, in that one area, we seem to be drawing closer together.

### It sounds like the decision to see a chiropractor is really up to me.

Yes, it is. If you get benefit and consider the treatment worth the expense, you are on your way. But don't be frightened into going by stories that your back is dangerously out of alignment or that your internal organs are at risk. Don't be threatened by the jargon discussed in Chapter 7. "Multiple subluxation complexes," one of my chiropractic favourites, translates as "several places in your spine where the joints are still in place but not quite and the whole thing seems very complicated."

Your reason for going is to feel better. If you are already feeling good, why go? If you don't get the results you want, why continue? I remember one caller to an open-line radio program who told me that she had been seeing her chiropractor every week for two years but there had been no change in her back pain. Her question to me was: "Should I keep going?" I am seldom at a loss for words, but on that occasion, I really had nothing to say.

### What about seeing a physiotherapist?

In many respects, seeing the physiotherapist is similar to seeing the chiropractor. The therapist generally puts stronger emphasis on either the use of self-directed exercise or passive pain-relieving devices they call modalities. Many physiotherapists take additional training in manual techniques and can provide both mobilization and manipulation of the spine. Chiropractors also make use of passive treatments, so the distinction between the two groups tends to blur.

### How do you become a physiotherapist?

Applicants to physiotherapy programs must have completed a four-year undergraduate degree at university. To become a physiotherapist requires two years of post-graduate training. The course includes the usual elements of anatomy and physiology, with particular emphasis on hands-on therapy and modality use. Upon completion, the successful candidate is awarded a Master's of Physical Therapy (MPT) degree. Although in this book we are talking about physiotherapists as spine specialists, many physiotherapists do not do spine work at all. They may focus on rehabilitation of other musculoskeletal complaints, or on neurological or respiratory problems.

### Would a physiotherapist be my best choice?

In most jurisdictions, physiotherapists are now allowed to provide primary care. That means you do not require a medical referral to see one. The majority of patients, however, still come on the recommendation of a doctor. Physiotherapists do not receive the training in diagnostic techniques that is part of a conventional medical curriculum. They do not have access to the investigational tools, including X-ray, that both the chiropractor and medical doctor can employ.

Some of the conditions physiotherapists identify and treat are not accepted by most doctors. One prime example is attributing low back pain to a small muscle, the piriformis, which arises on the inside of the pelvis, passes out through a notch at the back, and attaches near the base of the neck of the thigh bone. The tendon of piriformis has a smaller diameter than your little finger. It acts, along with several other muscles, to turn your leg outward. Because of the bony contours of your thigh bone and pelvis and because of the large buttock muscles that lie on top of it, the piriformis cannot be felt from the surface.

Many therapists believe that piriformis is a cause of back pain and that its action can irritate the sciatic nerve. They support the claim by locating an area of tenderness using heavy pressure on the buttock. Treatment is a series of stretching exercises. From the surgeon's perspective, the piriformis is only one of a number of muscles that work in concert at the back of the hip and cannot be isolated by palpation. Its action cannot affect the sciatic nerve, and its location makes it an extremely unlikely candidate to contribute to back pain. Piriformis syndrome exists in the minds of the physiotherapists, but is not recognized by the surgeon, even during surgery.

This sort of disagreement is apparent for several other anatomical locations. Many therapists and chiropractors believe it is possible to detect abnormal movement of the small spinal joints by feeling the back. As a spine surgeon, I have the opportunity of viewing these structures directly and I can see no way in which the slight movement of a joint that lies several centimetres below skin, fat, fibrous tissue, and tense muscle can be detected from the surface. The facet joints along the spine are about as prominent as the knuckles on your hand, but they are closer together. Try feeling the individual knuckles on the back of someone else's hand through a small stack of towels. Try to identify the joint movement if they gently wiggle one finger. Not possible.

**It sounds like you and the physiotherapists don't get along.**
Actually, we get along quite well. I rely heavily on their skills for the treatment of my neck and back patients. There are certainly things about which we disagree. I am not prepared to accept that any manual technique can detect abnormal movement in a single spinal joint. Nor do I accept that it can selectively increase the range of one joint while holding all the others completely still. I am happy to concede that a skilled physiotherapist can mobilize or manipulate discrete areas of the spine. More importantly, this manipulation can be very helpful in the management of acute neck and back pain.

In a broader sense, we are both working to achieve the same goals: speedy pain relief and a prompt return to normal activity. Our understanding of the underlying processes may be different, and our methods may vary, but together we make an effective team. I am much less concerned about the exact source of the problem than about how it can be clinically identified and properly managed. There is only one area where our differing philosophies give me concern. Physiotherapists with a passion for manual techniques concentrate on affecting small movements within the spine to such an extent that they convey to the patient a sense that the back is so delicately balanced and so fragile that even the smallest ill-conceived movement could spell disaster. Creating that groundless fear is right up there with promoting the slipped disc.

### Is there such a thing as a standard physiotherapy treatment?

No, there isn't. The term physiotherapy is as poorly defined and as all-encompassing as the term medicine. When patients tell me that their back was treated with physiotherapy, I have no idea exactly what they mean. They might as well tell me that they treated their problem by taking pills. The information is too vague to help.

Physiotherapists can be broadly divided into two groups; those who advocate a passive approach, including pain-relieving modalities and hands-on therapy, and those who advocate an active regime, including patient education and exercise training. Most therapists will combine both aspects. I favour placing the emphasis on the active portion.

A number of individual therapists have developed particular routines and techniques that bear their name. These special approaches are generally taught in a series of instructional courses and gather devoted followers. Proponents of the different methods often strenuously disagree with each other. Physiotherapists are anything but a homogeneous group.

### What sort of treatments for my back/neck can I expect to receive from a physiotherapist?

You may get manual therapy, back education, exercises, and instructions for your daily routines. Most of the other treatments will come from a variety of modalities and special techniques. Many of these are also available from chiropractors.

Some modalities, like hot and cold packs, are not much different from the sort of thing you can apply yourself. In fact, there is no difference in the depth of heat penetration from a hot water bottle and a professionally applied hot pack. Physiotherapists use a great deal of electrical stimulation. Nearly 90 per cent of all transcutaneous electric nerve stimulation (TENS) applications are carried out by physiotherapists. TENS is believed to trigger the gate mechanism in the spinal cord and block transmission of the patient's typical pain. TENS units may be used in the clinic or taken home by the patient for self-directed use. Its big brother is a machine that delivers interferential current. This device is only available in a professional setting. The electrical stimulus is delivered through lubricated sponges or suction cups. It too acts to close the spinal gate and block the patient's pain. Its theoretical advantage is that it can deliver different electrical waveforms that prevent the body from adapting to the therapeutic current, thereby circumventing the body's attempts to keep the gates open. It's rather like rotating the shield harmonics on the Starship *Enterprise*.

Another staple of the physiotherapists' passive arsenal is ultrasound, which is a professionally directed microwave. Delivered in a pulsed fashion, it is claimed to have an anti-inflammatory effect. In a continuous mode, it is a heat-delivery system, like heating a cup of coffee in the microwave oven.

Although they all have been used for many years and have been the subject of numerous investigations, the method of action for all these standard modalities remains speculative. None has ever been shown to produce clinical improvement in a consistent, statistically valid manner.

## What about some of the other modalities, like cold laser therapy?

The word laser stands for light amplification by stimulated emission of radiation. The laser beam possesses two important characteristics. First, it is highly columnated, which means it can travel over great distances without separating. That finely focused quality allows CD players to read the discs, and it is why surveyors use lasers to lay out roads. The beam's second property is coherence. That means that the units of light energy, the photons, move together in unison rather than radiating out randomly. This highly structured pattern allows the laser beam to develop enormous amounts of energy. You see this in the demonstrations in science museums where the laser burns a hole through a brick.

Lasers come in different classes, depending upon the strength of the beam. The laser found in the physiotherapy clinic has a very low energy level, hence its name "cold laser." It is not capable of burning anything except, perhaps, the retina of your eye, if improperly used. It has the potency of the laser pointer I use in my lectures. Employing a cold laser to treat spinal pain overlooks one very important fact. When that low-intensity laser beam strikes the skin, it is diffused, and within a few millimetres, it is no longer coherent or columnated. It is simply a beam of red (or green or yellow) light. If you believe that coloured light will help your pain, you can save the time and expense of a professional visit by buying a coloured light bulb at the hardware store and shining it on your back.

Laser therapy is an excellent example of the problems that we face with the increasing technology that surrounds back and neck care. It is certainly a high-tech device, but it doesn't do any good.

### Why, then, do patients insist that the laser helped their back?

Two reasons. First, neck and back pain are prone to frequent, spontaneous remissions. Many times the pain just goes away, sometimes for months or years. Second is the placebo effect: the body's response to a treatment you expect will be helpful. The placebo effect is real. The pain relief is genuine. The process appears to be based within the neural transmitting system of the brain, and we have already seen how powerful that can be. The placebo effect is widely thought to occur in about 30 per cent of patients receiving a sham treatment. New research has suggested that the number may be closer to twice that percentage. When you consider the combination of a history of frequent, spontaneous recovery and a strong belief in a useless therapy, it is easy to see why the laser and so many other modalities have gained reputations they do not deserve.

### But you said if it feels good it is good for you!

I still believe that. But a placebo, like the classic sugar pill, need not be expensive. And because it is only a placebo, its effects cannot be predicted and are not consistent. I have no objection to taking advantage of the benefit when it occurs, but I don't believe placebo response should be the basis for a treatment protocol.

I was talking about the role of modalities with a physiotherapist. He recalled an embarrassing situation from his early days in practice. His patient was scheduled to have ultrasound for neck pain. He was running late and the lubricating jelly was missing. He found an old tube, but it had a hole in it, and it squirted all over his hands and the patient's neck. By the time he had cleaned up the mess and finally began treatment, he was further behind than ever. Then, to make a bad day even worse, the patient had a severe reaction to the ultrasound therapy. She became flushed and dizzy and thought she might pass out. The therapist immediately reached to turn the unit off and found that he had never turned it on. The patient had not received any ultrasound. She had received no treatment at all except for the placebo that, in this case, made her sick.

## What about acupuncture? Is that a placebo?

There may be some placebo effect, but there appears to be something more. Acupuncture is not difficult to learn. Some physiotherapists and chiropractors use acupuncture after having been trained in a few professional-education seminars. At least one university in Canada offers a full course for those who wish to pursue the technique in greater detail.

Acupuncture seems to release chemicals within the brain that interfere with the processing of the pain signal. It appears to be a legitimate analgesic, but like any analgesic, its effect varies from person to person. Two things are clear. Acupuncture's effect in a chronic situation is much less impressive than when it is used in acute pain. And acupuncture is only a pain-control technique. It causes no changes in the structure, function, or state of wear within the spine.

## Does craniosacral therapy work like acupuncture?

I do not believe craniosacral therapy works at all except as a placebo. It is based on several highly suspect premises. An osteopathic student proposed the fundamental theory in the early 1900s. He hypothesized that since there are visible joint lines on the human skull, and since all of nature's designs have a purpose, movement must take place in these joints. The goals of craniosacral therapy are to alter the movement of the various parts of the skull and realign the body's "direction of energy." The theory states that normally your head expands and contracts several times each minute. When your head enlarges, your spine shortens (rather like the balloon dogs the clown makes at the fair). This head/spine cycle is the basis for the name craniosacral. With disease, the rhythm is disrupted, and treatment is intended to correct the imbalance.

None of these things actually occur. The bones of the skull in the adult are firmly bonded together and no movement is possible. Your head cannot enlarge or contract. In any case, your spine is not attached to the skull in a way that would allow any skull movement to be transmitted. The idea of "direction of energy" remains totally unproven.

Craniosacral therapy works, if it works at all, because of the placebo effect, and because the treatment consists of having your scalp massaged for twenty minutes while you lie in a relaxed, comfortable position. I know one craniosacral therapist who spends this time helping you talk over the stresses of your daily life. It sounds pleasant and it may be helpful, but it has nothing to do with rearranging the bones in your skull.

Like so many of these marginal treatments, the claims for craniosacral therapy are extensive. Its proponents allege it can be used to treat everything from allergies to mental retardation. These sorts of claims prey on vulnerable patients, and that is taking the placebo effect too far.

### What about reflexology and magnets and copper bracelets and ...?

The list does go on. Most of these agents have no scientific validity, yet all possess rabid supporters. My niece has completed a two-year program of reflexology. Some years ago she used it to treat my toothache. To my complete amazement, the pain in my face almost disappeared for a short while. I have no idea why it worked. I am sure it is not because she drew the evil humours of my body through my toes, as she told me she was doing. But the fact remains that I had a short respite from the pain. Do I recommend reflexology for my patients with neck pain? No, I don't. I realize we don't have all the answers, but I cannot condone treatments that make claims with no scientific basis or that mislead back- and neck-pain sufferers.

Magnetic therapy is supposed to induce electrical charges within the tissues by placing them inside a magnetic field. One brochure promotes it as a treatment for everything from headaches to haemorrhoids. There are heated discussions about whether the benefits are better if all the magnets are facing in the same direction or if the magnetic poles are mixed. And there is absolutely no proof that it does anything at all. A podiatrist friend of mine had a magnetic ring on the floor in his office to treat foot pain. It didn't work, but he left it there for the amusement of watching patients dip their toe into the circle and quickly pull it back out of fear that the magnetic field would dissolve their foot. Foolish, perhaps, but that is the power of misunderstood technology.

## I know you are not impressed with computerized traction. Why not?

Applying traction with the aid of a computer to analyse the stresses on the spine does not change the fact that pulling on your back can give, at best, temporary relief. Claims that traction with the computer can somehow improve the nourishment of the disc or reverse the natural ageing process are not true. But both of these claims were contained in a letter sent to one of my patients, who had requested information on the technique. I noticed that a larger proportion of the letter was devoted to explaining the cost structure for the twenty treatments (there's a discount if you prepay) and to the ways that the cost of the treatment might be made palatable to your insurance company or the tax department. Even after offloading part of the cost, the series of treatments costs nearly $3,000. I think that's way too much to pay for traction.

When computer-assisted traction was first introduced in my area, the traction was accompanied by three other treatment components. One was a ten-head laser that presumably could magnify the effect of a single cold laser by a factor of ten. The second was a water massage bed. It was a large metal cylinder looking vaguely like an MRI machine or the old "iron lung." You lay inside covered with a plastic sheet while a track in the lid allowed a water spray to move up and down over your body. The third additional treatment was the application of local anaesthetic patches over the sore spots in your neck and back. I have talked to several patients who attended for treatment but I have yet to find one who gained any lasting benefit. Not that I would have expected them to.

The effect of traction is temporary and so is the benefit of an anaesthetic patch. The ten-head laser magnified a non-effect. The waterbed may have felt strange, but it did nothing at all.

### I saw an infomercial about using electrical simulation to strengthen my abdominal muscles. Does that work?

Electrical muscle stimulation devices have been around a long time, and I can remember at least three periods in my practice when they gained popularity. Each time, they faded away (probably because they don't work) or were removed from the market. Electrical stimulation has a role in some types of neuromuscular rehabilitation but it cannot replace the effect of regular exercise on your muscles. It will not produce weight loss, increase strength, or create an athletic physique with well-defined abs. If you want to get in shape you will have to work for it. There is no free lunch.

Another electrical device sometimes used is surface electromyography (EMG). This is a variation of a machine that doctors use for electrodiagnosis. When applied to the skin surface with sticky pads, the EMG equipment can read some of the electrical activity in the muscles below. A few clinicians feel these devices are helpful in training people to relax tight back muscles by providing both visual and auditory biofeedback.

### Where do the kinesiologist and the registered massage therapist come in?

Kinesiology is a four-year undergraduate university degree. Students enter directly from high school. The focus of their training is body mechanics and movement. You can find kinesiologists working in a number of areas frequently associated with fitness clubs or exercise programs. CBI employs a large number of kinesiologists who work with the physiotherapists to establish active treatment programs. They also supervise patients who progress to fitness training.

A course in registered massage therapy (RMT) takes two years, and is generally run through a community college. Massage therapy is one of the fastest-growing alternative treatments for neck and back pain. There are a few studies that suggest massage may be as beneficial to the sore back and neck as mobilization or manipulation. It certainly feels good and, so far at least, it seldom makes exaggerated claims. I think it must be human nature for some practitioners to exaggerate their talents. One massage therapist told me that she was able to feel the heat from an inflamed nerve right through the sheet. Another massage therapist declared that by massaging a client's neck, he could feel when one of the discs was ready to let go. Those sorts of nonsensical statements can only detract from the value of a simple and safe method of short-term pain relief.

### When should I see an osteopath?

Andrew Taylor Still founded the first school of osteopathy in 1892. Osteopathic medicine differs from conventional medical thinking through its increased emphasis on manipulative therapy. Educational requirements to become a Doctor of Osteopathy (DO) are much the same as those for becoming an MD. Both require an undergraduate degree followed by four years of medical training.

Osteopaths often take further specialty training, frequently in the same facilities that train medical specialists. In the United States, where osteopathy was founded, osteopaths are licensed to perform the same services as general practitioners. They treat such non-skeletal conditions as kidney disease and high blood pressure. Although many retain the emphasis on manual therapy gained from their training, a practising DO may be indistinguishable from a practising MD.

In other countries, there are differing restrictions on the services osteopaths are allowed to provide. In Canada, osteopaths are licensed as chiropractors and are allowed to practise only drugless therapy. An osteopath can manipulate or adjust your spinal joints and may administer

physical treatments of the same sort offered by the chiropractor and physiotherapist. But like both these practitioners, he or she is allowed to offer
you only non-prescription medication, such as vitamin pills.

For osteopaths who practise only manual medicine, my comments are
much the same as those for the physiotherapist and the chiropractor. But no
profession can be painted in such broad strokes. Each contains exemplary
practitioners and each has, I am sure, members of whom it is less proud.

### Which medical doctors should I consider seeing for my neck or back problems?

There are several medical specialties that take a particular interest in spinal
problems. Although they each have a different perspective, they are all able
to order the necessary investigations and prescribe medication when
required. They all take additional training after completing a medical degree.

The physiatrist approaches back and neck problems in a manner similar
to the physiotherapist. In most hospitals, the physiatrists and physiotherapists are both attached to a department of rehabilitation medicine. Like
physiotherapists, physiatrists train in the management of a wide spectrum
of musculoskeletal conditions, and many develop specialty interests that do
not include the spine. A consultation with a physiatrist often leads to a prescription for specific physiotherapy treatments or mechanical therapy.

A rheumatologist deals primarily with the medical management of diseases in the musculoskeletal system. Since many of these disorders affect
the spine, rheumatologists have an interest in spinal problems. But their
focus is not usually on the common mechanical complaints that affect
most spine sufferers. A consultation with a rheumatologist may help to
rule out systemic conditions or to initiate investigations of possible underlying non-mechanical causes of back or neck pain.

A neurologist deals primarily with diseases and disorders of the nervous
system. Although they are sometimes involved in cases of acute Pattern 3
sciatica or the neurogenic claudication of Pattern 4, much of their practice
is centred on conditions like multiple sclerosis, meningitis, or stroke.

Psychiatrists and psychologists may become involved with neck
and back pain as they relate to a patient's emotional well-being or altered

behaviour. The potential problem is that, by training, both these specialties tend to see a wider range of possible personality disorders or psychiatric illnesses than might be apparent to the physiatrist, rheumatologist, or spine surgeon. This is not necessarily a good thing. Missing a psychiatric or psychological diagnosis could certainly misdirect treatment, but becoming overly involved in the patient's mental problems can easily divert attention from an underlying, easily correctable mechanical disorder.

A few psychiatrists and psychologists take a special interest in pain. Even fewer take an interest in the patterns of disability behaviour so commonly associated with spinal disorders. And I know from personal experience that referring a depressed patient with back pain to a general psychiatrist can be a frustrating experience. I saw a woman for Pattern 4 symptoms. Her major complaint to me was the fact that her leg pain stopped her from ballroom dancing. I initiated an active treatment program and measured her progress with periodic reviews of her pain-free walking distance. Her therapy produced a substantial improvement not only in her ability to walk but also in her associated low back pain. But in spite of her progress, she did not return to her dancing. One day after my assessment, and in the face of my obvious pleasure in her improvement, she confided to me that the main reason she had not gone back to dancing was that she and her husband were experiencing serious marital difficulties. She was simply too depressed and too upset to participate.

Since I had reached the limit of my ability to help, I referred her to a psychiatrist, in the hopes that he could find some way of improving her mental state. She saw him only once. I received a consultation report informing me that he would be unable to help because this woman had back pain. He had arranged for her to see a spine surgeon.

## Does that sort of poor communication happen often?

Perhaps not to that degree, but it certainly does occur. Medical specialists tend to look at problems in a very compartmentalized way. If a particular condition doesn't fit their area of expertise, they may not know what to do with it.

One of my favourite examples is the tug of war that takes place between the spine surgeon and the vascular surgeon over the patient with Pattern 4 leg pain. The pain of neurogenic claudication is caused by insufficient blood flow to the nerves in the spine. Almost identical symptoms can occur in the legs as a result of poor blood flow to the muscles themselves. To make matters more complicated, some patients can have both.

Let's assume that the consultation starts with the spine surgeon, who recognizes the claudication pain pattern. He can find no convincing evidence of a narrowed spinal canal to account for the symptoms. As part of his investigation, he sends the patient to a vascular surgeon. The vascular surgeon identifies the same pattern of pain, but cannot locate a sufficient narrowing in the blood vessels to guarantee that it is the cause.

The patient is in trouble, and both surgeons have some reason to suspect that the problem is in their territory. Neither has absolute proof. Something has to be done and someone will have to operate. Each surgeon would prefer that the other operate first. If the operation is a success, everyone looks good, but if it fails to solve the problem, the second surgeon gets to step in and save the day.

By odd coincidence, I had just finished writing this chapter when I received a letter from a vascular surgeon regarding a mutual patient with severe neurogenic claudication. The consultation concludes, "Although he has significant vascular disease, improvement of this vascular disease will not improve his symptoms entirely. He needs a multidisciplinary approach. It may be that attending to his spinal stenosis and symptoms of sciatica prior to vascular surgery would be the most efficacious approach." I guess it's my turn to go first.

### Besides the vascular surgeon, are there any other surgical specialties that might take an interest in the spine?

Urologists sometimes get involved because of the back pain that occurs with a kidney stone or because of the referred genital pain that can accompany Patterns 1 and 2.

## What about a more holistic approach?

Holistic medicine is portrayed by many of its practitioners as a major departure from common practice. In fact, it just represents good medicine. Its practitioners and advocates imply that no other doctors pay attention to the entire patient. The rest of us are accused of merely treating specific complaints as though they were isolated from the rest of the person.

A good spine surgeon can never ignore the rest of the patient. To be a good spine surgeon, you must first be a good back doctor. Pain is far too intimately involved with stress and emotion for you to ignore the patient's mental state. Back and neck pain can be caused by such widely divergent problems as job dissatisfaction or a benign bone tumour. The one should be dealt with through counselling and changes in the workplace; the other demands surgery. The spine surgeon who fails to take into account the patient's circumstances, or who fails to recognize the devastating emotional impact of a failed spinal procedure, cannot deliver good spine care.

The concept of holistic medicine grew as a reaction to the increasing specialization of medicine. The holistic practitioner was supposed to be interested not only in your head cold and backache but in your children's performance at school and how you are getting on at work as well. Looked at in that way, the perfect example of a holistic doctor is a competent and caring family physician.

The holistic approach also appears to answer the patient's desire to see a specialist, since many patients perceive the holistic doctor to have had special training. But holistic medicine is not actually specialty medicine. Seeing a holistic doctor cannot replace a consultation with an expert in a specific field. I hear from many family doctors that their opinion is no longer valued and that, as far as they can tell, their patients visit them only to obtain a referral to an expert. As a consequence, most spine specialists see a lot of patients who do not require their advanced expertise. Meanwhile, patients who do need special consideration find it harder to get an appointment and are forced to wait longer.

This same emphasis on dealing with the whole patient has come to be called wellness. Medical consultants are perceived to treat only sick people, while this new breed of physician keeps them well. It sounds good but when you think about it, managing your illness effectively brings about the same result. It leaves you feeling well.

Holistic medicine should not be confused with homeopathy. They are completely different. Homeopathy is a system of medicine based on the Law of Similars. This law is a two-hundred-year-old theory that the best way to cure a problem is to stimulate the body to heal itself. A commonly used example is treatment of the common cough. Homeopathy considers that the symptoms, no matter how uncomfortable, represent the body's attempt to restore itself to health. Instead of looking upon the symptoms as something wrong that must be set right, homeopathy sees them as signs of the way the body is attempting to recover. So instead of trying to stop the cough, as conventional medicine would do, homeopathy provides a remedy that will cause a cough in a healthy person and thus stimulate the ill body to restore itself. I am not an expert in homeopathy, but the thought of taking something to aggravate my typical Pattern 1 back pain so that I will get better just does not appeal to me.

Homeopathy is practised by chiropractors, veterinarians, dentists, nurse practitioners, and acupuncturists. There are osteopaths, and the occasional medical doctor, who use the techniques as well.

The group most frequently associated with homeopathy is the naturopaths. Naturopathy is a broader but distinct system of non-invasive health care that uses neither surgery nor drugs. The naturopath relies on education, counselling, and natural substances to gain benefit. They make wide use of food extracts, vitamins, minerals, air, water, heat, cold, sound, light, magnetic therapy, homeopathic preparations, and exercise. Although I do not subscribe to the approach, I can certainly agree that education and exercise are important aspects of managing low back and neck pain.

## Is there anyone else?

Yes, the spine surgeon. At the moment, there are two kinds. Some spine surgeons are neurosurgeons. Their training, in addition to spine work, focuses on trauma and tumours in the brain. They tend to regard the spine as a structure that gets in the way, as it encases the nerves. Their surgeries are generally for spinal-cord or nerve tumours, or for the acute nerve-root involvement that produces sciatica or arm-dominant pain in Pattern 3. They also open the spinal canal to treat the nerve compression of Pattern 4.

The other group of spine surgeons trains as orthopaedic surgeons. They tend to see the spine as a mechanical structure full of moving parts and linking joints. The nerves are something that get in the way and must be protected as the surgeon stabilizes or replaces the worn discs, which generate back- or neck-dominant pain.

It has been standard practice in many centres for both the neurosurgeon and the orthopaedic surgeon to operate on the same spine. The neurosurgeon removes what is necessary to solve the problem and the orthopaedic surgeon stabilizes what is left so that it remains mechanically sound. That dichotomy is closing. Newly trained spine surgeons are comfortable dealing with both the neurological and the biomechanical elements of the spine. Training programs once populated by a single specialty now accommodate both. Orthopaedic surgeons can deal with pathology in the nerves and neurosurgeons can fuse the spine. I see the time when the distinction between the neurosurgical and the orthopaedic spine surgeon will be gone and, like today's hand surgeon, the specialty training and not the prior experience will be what matters.

### As a back doctor and a spine surgeon, how do you investigate a patient referred to you with long-standing neck or back pain?

I begin with a thorough history and the appropriate physical examination. In most cases, they will be enough to identify the pattern of mechanical neck or back pain and allow me to proceed with an initial treatment routine. Further investigation is not necessary during the first few weeks of an attack. Many of the people I see have already had X-rays and special studies. They are frequently surprised to see how little the studies assist me in making my preliminary diagnosis.

I pay special attention to anything in the history or the physical examination that might suggest a serious medical problem or possibility of malignancy. But I start by identifying the common mechanical patterns. I believe that focusing on pain-pattern recognition makes my job easier.

Over 90 per cent of the patients I see can be correctly placed into one of the four patterns. That leaves me free to concentrate my energy and my diagnostic efforts on the few remaining cases that cannot be categorized.

### If you do investigate, what tests do you use?

The first steps are usually basic bloodwork and X-ray studies.

By analysing your blood, the medical laboratory can tell me a great deal about your general state of health, the presence of infection, or the possibility of a malignancy. The tests would include your haemoglobin, a measure of the number of red cells in your blood and, indirectly, of the iron in your body. Low haemoglobin reduces the blood's oxygen-carrying capacity. It raises the possibility of a number of chronic diseases. An old test, but one that is still useful, is the erythrocyte sedimentation rate (ESR). It measures the speed with which the blood cells clump together, and has long been known to be a marker of inflammation somewhere in the body. It is completely non-specific, but it can be very helpful. Along with another general marker of inflammation, the C-reactive protein, the ESR is still one of the best ways for the lab to detect an infected disc. This is a rare but potentially serious cause of non-mechanical back pain.

Other blood tests include screening for rheumatoid arthritis, ankylosing spondylitis, and a number of other generalized inflammatory diseases. Bloodwork may also include tests of your liver function, a measure of your prostatic enzymes, and a check of several specific elements, minerals, and hormones.

A urinalysis may be helpful in discovering kidney disease or certain types of spinal malignancy.

Sooner or later, virtually every spine patient gets a set of plain X-rays. They are of remarkably little help in identifying the sources of mechanical back and neck pain, but are mandatory when investigating a serious spinal injury. Fractures and even dislocations of the spine can be missed on the physical examination. But the trauma that requires an X-ray is a serious injury like falling off a roof, not bending over to put on your socks.

An X-ray is produced by a single beam of electrons striking a sensitized surface, producing X-ray radiation. The image owes its appearance to the fact that X-rays are stopped more readily by the bone than by the soft tissues. As a result, the bones appear white and everything else goes a darker shade of grey or black. Anything that fails to block the X-rays cannot be seen. A plain X-ray cannot reveal the location of nerves or individual muscles. It cannot see discs, and it certainly cannot identify inflammation. Yet I know that patients are told their X-ray has revealed an inflamed bulging disc. I wish it were so easy.

Typical of the misunderstanding and needless fear created by erroneous interpretations of the pictures is an e-mail I received from a woman who was convinced she was "falling apart" because her doctor had told her the X-rays showed "sclerosis, slipping discs at T10 and T11, deterioration, inflammation in the lower lumbar with osteoarthritis, and the beginnings of osteoporosis." Sclerosis means the bone is more dense than usual. The extra material stops more electrons and the X-ray appears whiter. The thickened bone is a natural response to wear and it produces no pain. Discs never slip, and they can't be seen on the X-ray anyway. Neither can inflammation. Deterioration and osteoarthritis are merely the signs of normal ageing. Plain X-rays cannot detect the beginnings of osteoporosis; over half the bony material must be gone before any change is visible on the X-ray. This woman's X-rays showed nothing except that her spine was as old as she was.

X-rays cast a shadow in only one direction. A single view of the spine is usually of little help. It may offer no more information than looking at the edge of a postcard. Multiple views are required. Because X-rays are created at a single point, the beam should be positioned directly in front of the area of the spine to be assessed. The further away you move from the point of origin, the more the image is distorted. Modern X-ray techniques have greatly reduced the patients' exposure to dangerous radiation. Spine X-rays are safe. They just aren't all that helpful.

People are always surprised to learn that there is no correlation between the amount of degenerative change seen on X-ray and the amount of back pain they suffer. With the exception of spondylolisthesis, where there is a limited connection, all the other changes of narrowed discs, knobby joints, or bone spurs cannot be directly translated into the patient's symptoms.

## Is that where the CT scan comes in?

The CT, or CAT, scan is another form of X-ray. CAT stands for computer-ized axial tomography. The term tomography refers to the process of taking a series of X-rays. Tomography has been around a long time, but now it is rarely used without the aid of the computer. The images on the sensitized surface are viewed by the computer rather than recorded on X-ray film. A series of X-ray slices is obtained so that the spine can be viewed one slice at a time. As the technique of CT has improved, the thick-ness of the slices has decreased. Now, it is possible to look at X-ray sections of the back and neck that are no more than a couple of millimetres apart.

The X-ray image is the result of the radiation being absorbed differently by different structures. While the human eye might see no difference in the projected shadow, the computer can separate even slight variations in shading. It then enhances the differences, just as photographs taken in outer space are enhanced. With the computer's help, you can identify differences in density between the open space within the spinal canal and the nerve sac containing the cauda equina. Individual nerves become visible. A CT can show a bulging disc and the way it distorts the path of the nerve passing by. But it cannot show inflammation, and it certainly cannot reveal pain. About 30 per cent of the abnormalities it identifies are irrele-vant findings with no bearing on the patient's problem.

Occasionally, CT is combined with a myelogram. Myelography is a study in which an X-ray-opaque material is injected into the nerve sac within the spinal canal. Sixty years ago, myelography was the only way to identify pressure on the nerve sac. The myelogram would reveal indenta-tions that were assumed to be the result of something pressing in from outside the sac. Today, the myelogram is used to enhance the CT's view of the exiting nerves. Adding the X-ray marker makes the job of tracking the nerve's course easier. Since the bulging disc is also visible, a more accurate diagnosis is possible. CT-myelograms are particularly helpful in Pattern 4, where the canal is narrow and grossly distorted, and there may be several levels at which the nerves are being compressed.

## Is the MRI just a more accurate X-ray?

Magnetic resonance imaging, or MRI, is not an X-ray at all. Although the pictures look the same, they are very different. An MRI is the computer's representation of the location and amount of hydrogen in your body. Since body hydrogen is bound as water ($H_2O$), the MRI records the relative moisture of the body's structures.

The image is obtained by placing the subject in a large electromagnet. The magnetic field lines up the body's molecules in one direction, much the same way iron filings line up with the poles of a bar magnet. Once all the molecules are facing in the same direction, a radio signal is passed through the subject's body. The energy from the signal pushes the molecules out of alignment. As they resume their positions along the magnetic lines, the extra energy is retransmitted as small electrical signals. Each type of molecule sends a signal on a different frequency. Since hydrogen is plentiful, and since its signal is loud, it is the best voice for the computer to monitor. The location of the body's water also happens to be very important in the diagnosis of several spinal problems.

Because of the way the picture is created, the MRI shows the bones as black (they are very dry) and the fluid within the spinal canal as white. Because young discs are largely water, a young disc is very light. As it ages and dries out, it becomes progressively darker. A dark disc is a dry disc, presumably one that has undergone extensive ageing and wear.

Because inflammation includes an accumulation of fluid, it shows up easily on an MRI. Because so many malignant tumours contain large amounts of water, they too can be quickly identified. But just like the CT, the MRI cannot view pain. What is more troubling is the fact that two-thirds of the abnormal findings obtained with this study have no direct correlation to the clinical symptoms in the neck or back. And because MRI is a computer-generated picture, its characteristics can be substantially changed by the computer's settings. Technical manipulation can alter the apparent size of a disc bulge or the amount of water that appears to be inside the disc.

Many people consider the MRI to be the final arbiter for the source of neck and back pain. It can't serve that function. Its studies are invaluable in the examination for spinal cancer and for assessing the bleeding, fluid collection, and nerve injury that follow major trauma. They are practically useless in assessing the source of simple mechanical neck or back pain.

**So except for tumours and trauma, do the MRI pictures help at all?**
The MRI, the CT, and the myelogram are all very helpful in preparation for surgery. As our surgical techniques become more precise and less invasive, it is essential that we know exactly where we are going before we start. The MRI can determine that. But these studies should be used to locate the problem after, and not before, the decision for surgery is made. They are road maps that lead to a precise destination. But you get a map because you want to take a trip. If you have no plans to leave home, seeing a map should not make you change your mind.

As an aid to diagnosis of mechanical back pain, MRIs can sometimes do more harm than good. I recently saw a woman whom I easily diagnosed as having Pattern 1 back-dominant pain. Her pain was intermittent and could easily have been controlled. I did my best to reassure her but my consultation did not include enough bells or whistles. She obtained an MRI on her own so that we could both discover what was really wrong with her back. Here is the interpretation of the MRI provided by the radiologist.

1. L1–L2: Small to moderate right paracentral to posterolateral disc herniation encroaching on the right foramen.
2. L2–L3: Moderate broad disc bulge.
3. L3–L4: Moderate to large left foraminal disc herniation compressing the exiting left L3 nerve root.
4. L4–L5: Moderate to large right paracentral to posterolateral disc herniation filling the right neural foramen and compressing the exiting right L4 nerve root and the L4 ventral aspect of the thecal sac.
5. L5–S1: Small focal right foraminal disc herniation abutting the exiting right L5 nerve root.

This woman had no symptoms of nerve-root irritation or nerve-root compression. Her mechanical back pain could be abolished easily with a few sloppy push-ups. The information on the MRI did nothing to solve the problem. She was most definitely not a surgical candidate. But after reading that report, there was no way that she was willing to believe my story. She left to find another surgeon who presumably would be willing to operate at all five levels of her lumbar spine, removing disc bulges and enlarging the exit canals on both sides of her back.

At least when she left my office, she was only frustrated, not frightened. It was a very different situation for the worried young husband who sent me an e-mail about his twenty-three-year-old wife. It read in part, "She has recently been diagnosed with three collapsed discs in her lower back. The surgeon who requested the MRI said that it would be too dangerous to operate. He referred her to a chronic pain clinic so that she can learn how to manage her pain, as she will have this problem for the rest of her life."

Magnetic resonance imaging may have condemned this woman to a lifetime of pain. That plaintive e-mail holds many lessons. Young, healthy women do not collapse three discs. Discs don't collapse; they slowly dry out. Surgery on worn discs in the low back is not dangerous: demanding, perhaps, but not dangerous. What the surgeon really meant was that he didn't want to operate. Surgery is not the answer. The solution is active exercise, education, and control. Instead, he offered her a clinic to focus on her symptoms. If he didn't plan to operate, why did the surgeon order the MRI? Seeing three dark discs may have destroyed this woman's life.

I don't operate on pictures. I operate on people. I tell my residents quite clearly that if the picture looks so terrible, they should take a pair of scissors and cut out all the bumps they can see. Just leave the patient alone.

### Are there any tests that *can* help?

No single test can reliably diagnose the causes of mechanical back and neck pain. A few may give me useful additional information.

One of the most controversial and painful is the discogram. Opinion is so polarized that some surgeons will not operate without seeing a discogram, while others consider performing the test to be malpractice.

The discogram is done by injecting an irritating, X-ray-blocking dye through a needle into the middle of the disc. X-rays will reveal the shape the fluid assumes, and whether or not it leaks out through cracks in the disc's outer shell. It is usually possible to distinguish between a young, moist disc and one that has dried out and whose outer shell has failed. Occasionally, a CT scan is used to further locate the exact position of the injected material.

But the appearance of the disc doesn't matter very much. Some clinicians believe it does not matter at all. Discography is designed to provoke pain. Injecting dye into the painful disc will reproduce typical Pattern 1 back-dominant pain. In fact, it may escalate the pain to a level the patient has never experienced before. The test is really no more sophisticated than saying, "Could you please stop screaming long enough to tell me if that hurt? It did? Well, I guess we've found your sore disc."

The trouble with discography is that sometimes apparently healthy discs hurt. And discs that look completely worn feel no pain. And when the pain is brought on by the test, it must be precisely the same pain as the one that the surgeon is hoping to eliminate. Discography is limited by the patient's ability to report the nature of the pain, by numerous potential flaws in the techniques, and by the presence of any pain-focused behaviour.

Discography may be helpful before surgery. It should never be used merely to investigate back or neck pain.

### That test sounds awful. Don't you have anything that hurts a little less?

Nerve-root injections and facet blocks both attempt to eliminate, not aggravate, the patient's typical pain. The theory assumes that if one facet joint is causing the problem and we can anaesthetize that particular joint, the pain will stop and we will have located the trouble. Similarly, if one of the exiting nerves is responsible for the spread of the pain into the arm or leg, freezing that nerve should temporarily eliminate the patient's symptoms and identify which level of the spine is involved.

The problem is that the joints receive nerve signals from more than one nerve. That collection of nerves also supplies the joint above and the joint below. Because the exiting nerve and the joint are so close together, it is very easy to accidentally anaesthetize the nerve and never know it. What the technician takes to be elimination of joint pain may actually be the result of anaesthetizing the adjacent neural tissue. And there is the definite possibility that neither the nerve nor the joint are the source of the trouble in the first place. A set of facet or nerve blocks may not hurt very much, but they may not help very much either.

### My mother had a bone scan. What is that?

A bone scan is a reading of the levels of radiation that appear in the different bones of your body after a radioactive material is injected into your blood stream. That sounds frightening, but the procedure is completely harmless and painless. The radioactive substance disappears rapidly. The pictures are taken shortly after the injection and, shortly after that, the injected material is completely gone. The radioactive substance used is one that incorporates into the bone. The scan detects the areas where the marker accumulates. These are areas where the bone is active and repairing itself. Scans will "light up" in areas where cancer is attacking the bone and the bone is fighting back, or in areas where the body is repairing the process of advanced maturity by growing bone spurs.

A different marker can be used. It targets the white blood cells, one of your body's first lines of defence against infection. The assumption is that if the scan sees a large collection of white cells, they are in located in an infected area.

A modern variation of the standard bone scan is called the SPECT scan. The letters stand for single-proton emission computerized tomography. Here, computerized tomography is used in conjunction with an injected radioactive marker. The SPECT scan does not replace a CT or an MRI, but it may be used to gain more information about the exact location of a problem.

### Do any of your tests look at things beside the physical structures?

It can be helpful to measure nerve impulses directly. A surgeon may assume that a nerve is malfunctioning because of problems in the spine. In reality, the trouble may be pressure on the nerve somewhere in the arm or leg. A common example is the difficulty sometimes encountered in deciding whether one of the nerves leading to the hand is being squeezed at the wrist, a condition called carpal tunnel syndrome, or whether the problem comes from pressure on the same nerve in the neck as a result of a bulging disc. The best way to tell may be to measure the electrical flow along the course of the nerve to locate the obstruction. It is exactly the same technique, on a much smaller scale, that the telephone repairperson uses to locate a break in the underground telephone line. We can do the same thing with the nerves using an electrical measuring device. The test is called a nerve conduction study, and it is performed by inserting extremely fine needles at several points along the length of the nerve. The test is uncomfortable but not painful. Taking readings at each level will allow us to locate the block.

A similar test using the same equipment is called electromyography. In this test, the nerve is stimulated and the effect is measured by fine needles inserted into the muscle. In addition to measuring the flow of nerve impulses, an EMG also examines the nerve's effect on the muscle and the activity of the muscle fibres themselves. This is a much more precise analysis of the muscle's action than that obtained by surface electrodes in biofeedback training.

An EMG may be helpful in separating true muscle weakness from unwillingness to move for fear of increasing pain. It can also tell us about the possibility or rate of recovery if there is a power loss after nerve compression in Pattern 3 or Pattern 4.

It is also possible to measure the speed of electrical conduction through the spinal cord. The measurements are called somatosensory evoked potentials (SSEP). While the subject's brain waves are being monitored, a sensory nerve in the arm or leg is stimulated. The character, size, and speed of the response give information about the function of the spinal cord. SSEP may monitor spinal-cord function during surgical procedures where the spinal cord is at risk, such as correction of severe scoliosis.

# CHAPTER TWELVE

## *You're Going to Cut* What?

You would think that with all the advances in surgical technique, spine surgeons could do just about anything by now. The truth is, we just keep on doing the same two things in a number of different ways. I believe that we are doing them better than we used to. There is no question that we are getting our patients back into action a lot faster. But sometimes making something more complicated or more technically advanced won't make it better.

Spine surgeons either remove pressure on the spinal cord or nerves or stabilize an area of mechanical failure. What they do has not changed, just how they do it. For seventy years we have recognized that bulging discs sometimes press on the nerves that pass across their surface. The resulting combination of pressure and inflammation produces the acute nerve irritation that causes Pattern 3 arm- or leg-dominant pain. For fifty years we have realized that increased bony growth within the spinal canal will compromise the blood supply to the nerves and produce leg pain typical of Pattern 4. The surgical answer in both cases is to remove the pressure. Whether this is done through a large open incision or whether it is performed through a tiny aperture with the aid of a microscope or television monitor, the surgical objective is the same: to eliminate pressure on the nerve.

For almost a hundred years we have observed the progressive mechanical deterioration that comes with age or the more sudden destruction that accompanies injury, infection, or tumour. The surgical solution has been to regain structural stability by joining one vertebra solidly to another. Whether we use wires or screws or plates or cages, the goal remains the same: to fuse the bones together.

Spine surgery has no place in any condition where the pain arises outside these two areas. The surgeon cannot make the spine better than before the nerve pressure or the mechanical deterioration began. Normal spines don't carry scars. The goal is to return patients to a normal life, but they go back with an altered spine.

Only one or two neck- and back-pain sufferers in a hundred are legitimate candidates for spinal surgery. While surgery's role is clear in major trauma or tumours invading the spine, it is far less obvious in the overwhelming majority of people who suffer mechanical neck and back pain. There is a wide divergence of opinion about what procedure, if any, will help. Decompression to release the pinched nerve in Pattern 3 or Pattern 4 has a reasonable probability of success. Of course, that implies the correct operation was done correctly and at the proper time.

But for those with back- and neck-dominant pain, the picture is cloudy indeed. Does a spinal fusion treat mechanical spine pain? Not consistently. And yet sometimes it succeeds. In spite of our impressive investigations, selecting the perfect surgical candidate remains as much an art as a science. In spite of our advanced techniques for surgery, the overall success rate has improved very little.

For spinal fusion, our expectations may be too high. The fused spine has lost part of its natural mobility and normal muscle has been replaced with scar. If back pain is the inevitable consequence of the human condition, then why should it be absent in a spine that has been subjected to surgery?

Perhaps we should more realistically aspire to a neck or back that only hurts some of the time, whose pain can be controlled with regular activity and simple adjustments to our daily lives. Perhaps the fused back should be exercised and strengthened as if it had never known the knife.

Exciting alternatives are over the horizon. Chemical moderators may eliminate pain and remove inflammation from a damaged nerve, rendering decompression obsolete. Fusions generated by genetic manipulation or the injection of bone-forming protein may eliminate the need for metallic fixation. But for now, we remain where we started: with surgical decompression and spinal fusion. They're not perfect. But they do work. I remember that every time I think of the young woman whose spine I fused for intractable mechanical low back pain. Now she says, "My back only hurts sometimes. When I catch air on my Harley."

## What's a decompression? It sounds simpler than fusion.

The commonest reason to perform a decompression is in order to remove part of a bulging disc that is causing Pattern 3 pain. We'll start there. The techniques for spinal decompression go by a number of different names. Patients are sometimes uncertain about what is planned because they don't realize that many of the procedures' names mean much the same thing.

The bony roof at the back of the spinal canal is called the lamina. Putting a hole in something is called an "otomy." Removing something entirely is called an "ectomy." If I put a hole in the lamina, I have performed a laminotomy. But since that hole has removed part of the lamina I have also performed a partial laminectomy. The two terms mean exactly the same thing. Consider surgery on the disc. If I cut a hole in the shell, I perform a discotomy (because the shell is called the annulus, the procedure can also be called an annulotomy). But I removed part of the disc when I cut my hole, so I also performed a partial discectomy. The three terms have the same meaning.

Many patients believe that disc surgery removes discs. It does not. Although we may extract portions of the central nucleus or even remove extensive sections of the outer shell, a large part of the disc remains. Spinal fusions extend around the disc or pass through its centre. Even the new artificial disc is located within the existing outer shell of the natural disc.

**So decompression is cutting holes in the bones and discs. What good does that do?**

Usually it exposes the nerves. A laminectomy (now I have removed the entire lamina) is only the first step in the decompression. Once I have taken the back off the spinal canal, the nerve sac and the exiting nerves are visible at the bottom of the hole. The bulging disc lies below that, and to get there, I must move the nerve and nerve sac out of the way.

**Isn't that dangerous?**

It's not dangerous, but it's certainly something that must be done with great care. Spine surgery requires a great deal of delicacy, but no more than might be expected of a watchmaker. Being a competent spine surgeon requires excellent technical skills. Still, I believe the greatest challenge is selecting the patients and the problems where surgery will produce a good clinical result.

Because the nerves in the low back have a long, sloping course, it is easier to move them aside in this region than it is to move the nerves in the neck. The cervical spinal canal also contains the spinal cord, which does not like to be moved at all. For that reason, a bulging disc in the neck is often approached from the front, with the surgeon reaching the spine by passing between the large blood vessels and the windpipe. As odd as it seems, the distance from the skin to the disc in the neck is about the same whether you enter from in front or behind.

**What happens when you reach the part of the disc that is pressing on the nerve?**

The pressure usually results from the protrusion of some of the fibrous material from inside the disc through a small rupture in the outer shell. People often think of the disc as a jelly-filled cushion, but the material doesn't look like jelly. I've tried many ways to describe it to patients and the best I can come up with is that rubbery lump of gristle you have left in your mouth after you've been chewing on a tough piece of meat for a while.

The bulge is under pressure and is usually covered by a thin membrane, the last remnant of the disc's outer shell. It looks like a large pimple.

When I cut the membrane with the tip of a small knife, the stringy material inside pushes out. I pick it up with my forceps and gently pull it out through that small hole. The piece is never large. It can be a fragment smaller than your small fingernail but never bigger than the whole tip of your little finger.

Once I have extracted the loose fragments of disc, I generally explore the area carefully with a fine hook to make sure there are no other pieces lurking in the corners. Some surgeons enlarge the original hole and use a tiny spoon to clean out any more loose pieces inside the disc. It's like cleaning out a pumpkin on a very small scale. If the disc rupture produced a very large rent, I will sometimes scrape the inside of the disc. Removing any additional loose pieces is intended to prevent them from sliding out later through the same hole and pinching the nerve again. It sounds like a good idea, but several studies have shown that scraping out the disc does not reduce the risk of recurrence. When the hole is quite small, and it usually is, I do not believe there is anything gained by making it larger. Once the fragment has been extracted, the operation is over.

### How long does it take?

That depends on how difficult it is to expose the disc and pull out the fragment. The nerves are surrounded by a collection of fine veins and I do my best not to tear one. A tear will do no permanent damage, but the bleeding can certainly slow you down. The operation can take anywhere from thirty minutes to a couple of hours, if things don't go as well.

### What can go wrong?

I prefer to talk about what can go right, but patients must be aware of the risks they run when they agree to undergo spine surgery. Outlining these risks and ensuring that the patient really understands the dangers is part of proper informed consent. My purpose in listing all the things that can go wrong is not to frighten the patient unnecessarily. I want to impress upon him or her that this is a major decision and one with potentially serious consequences. I generally start with the anaesthetic risk: everything from chipping a tooth to developing pneumonia. With modern techniques, there is less than one complication for every quarter of a million cases. Your chance of having serious trouble with the anaesthetic is about the same as your chance of being struck by lightning.

Any time I cut skin, there is a risk of infection. Any time I handle the nerves in your spine, there is a risk of nerve injury. The possibility of trouble is exceedingly low, but it can happen.

Your position on the operating table can interfere with the normal blood return from your legs. Some people develop inflammation and blood clots in their veins, complications called phlebitis and thrombosis. While this may not be serious, a portion of the clot can break loose and lodge in the lung. This complication, called pulmonary embolus, can be fatal. The position of your face must be checked carefully. Prolonged pressure on your eye can cause permanent damage.

Those are the major problems. Taken together, they occur in less than 3 per cent of spine surgeries. Most of the time, these complications can be managed successfully. But that doesn't make them any less serious.

There are even more things that can go wrong, not counting the possibility that the operating light breaks loose and falls from the ceiling. Operating through the disc in the low back puts me close to the great blood vessels behind the abdomen. Going a little too far could result in a serious vascular accident. There is even a remote chance of partial blindness unrelated to pressure on the eye. This may be caused by changes in the blood pressure in the brain, but no one really knows.

In the neck, additional risks include damage to the blood vessels that supply your brain; to your windpipe; to your oesophagus (the tube that runs from your throat to your stomach); to the spinal cord; or to the nerves that control either your vocal cords or your ability to swallow normally.

All these complications are rare. If your spine surgery is necessary, and the procedure carries a high rate of success, the risks are probably worth taking. But this is elective surgery, so the decision is up to you. I tell patients that spine surgery is not like having a haircut. Complications exist and some very nasty things can happen. If you don't like the result, you can't go back and ask for a trim to make things right.

## Neck surgery sounds very risky. How do you do a decompression in the neck?

Removing a portion of the disc in the neck can be done from behind in the same way I described for the low back. The main difference is that to avoid the spinal cord I come in more from the side by enlarging the exit hole where the nerve leaves the canal. Incidentally, that hole is called a foramen, and because I am making the hole bigger, the procedure is called a foraminotomy. Once I reach the disc and find the bulge, the procedure is no different than in the lumbar spine.

When I approach the neck from the front, I put a hole in the front of the disc and work my way through to the back removing the centre of the disc as I go. The deeper I get, the closer I come to the spinal cord. Eventually I reach the same membrane I see from the other side when I operate inside the canal. I attempt to extract as much of the protruding material, the chewed gristle, as I can, while still preserving that last remnant of the disc shell. I can remove it if I want, but I must be very careful so near the spinal cord.

When I approach the spinal canal from the front of the neck, I remove a lot of the disc. Although the space can be left open, most surgeons fill the centre of the disc with a plug of bone, usually taken from the crest of the patient's pelvis through a small cut in the skin over the hip. This bone will fuse into place and prevent any further movement at that level. The procedure has now become a discectomy – because so much of the disc has been taken out, "partial" is usually dropped – and fusion.

## When do you decide that surgery is necessary?

*I* don't decide. *We* do. The first step after you understand your problem and the risks involved with an operation is for you to agree that an operation is acceptable treatment. I will not order some investigations, like a CT myelogram, until after you have taken the decision to go ahead. Most patients with Pattern 3 get better without surgery. There is nothing to be lost by waiting except that you will have to endure the pain. Operating for acute sciatica is one of the few cases where the timing of the surgery is dictated by how much you hurt. If the pain is subsiding and you are prepared to put up with the pain that still remains, then I recommend we wait and see what nature can do.

Be very clear. Spine surgery is performed for the current problem, not for what might happen in the future. The surgeon should never operate "just in case." Done properly and for the right reasons, spine surgery can be very helpful. But it always carries risks, and it can lead to long-term difficulties. There is no purpose in accepting those negative consequences if there is no immediate problem to be solved. And spine surgery is not the treatment of last hope. It has its place and it has its time. Delaying the correct procedure past the point where it can be helpful is just as misguided as doing the wrong surgery right away.

People believe that surgery is more urgent if you develop weakness in the muscles supplied by the irritated nerve. In fact, the timing of the surgery does not seem to make a predictable difference. Many patients do recover their power immediately after the operation, but many others will regain full function without having any surgery at all. It is a factor to consider, but it should not force the decision and it does not dictate the timing. Muscles can recover after surgery even if we postpone the operation for several months.

The situation in the neck is the same. If anything, surgery can be delayed even longer. It is the amount of arm pain that is the deciding factor. Weakness in the arm muscles frequently recovers with or without the surgery. That recovery can occur more than a year after the pain began.

Once you have decided that an operation is worth the risk, the next decision is mine. I will carry out whatever investigations are necessary to convince myself that I am doing the right procedure at the right place for the right reason. No matter how much pain you report, if I cannot locate the exact site of the irritation, there is nothing I can do surgically.

### Does that ever happen?
It certainly does. There is one condition, a type of blood-vessel problem that affects the nerve root, that can look very much like Pattern 3 sciatica. But the problem is in the nerve's circulation and not from a bulging disc. This situation generally corrects itself within a couple of years. Those

months will be unpleasant but, as a surgeon with nothing to operate on, there is nothing surgical I can offer.

### If I decide I can't stand the pain and you can locate the trouble, what can I expect when I come to hospital?

In many cases, simple disc surgery is now done on an outpatient basis or as a short stay where you will go home within twenty-four hours. If the surgery is on your neck and I have had to add a fusion, things may go a little slower, but not much.

For posterior disc surgery, you do not require a brace and I don't impose any restrictions. Some surgeons are not quite as aggressive, but all of us agree that the sooner you start to move normally, the better it will be. You will be limited only by the soreness in your back. Since the surgery is done through a small incision with little disruption of the muscles, your back pain will subside rapidly. It should be no worse than the pain you might feel if you slipped and struck your back on the corner of the coffee table. The surgery hurts like a bad bruise because that's what it is.

If the operation is successful, your leg pain will be completely gone. Often, because of the remaining inflammation and post-surgical swelling, some of your original leg pain may return on the second or third day. This leg pain is intermittent and resolves rapidly as the swelling and inflammation disappear.

Recovering from spine surgery, like just about everything else in the world of neck and back pain, is a very personal thing. Your attitude and your expectations make a huge difference. I remember one patient, the owner of a clothing store, who had disc surgery the second week in December. A week later, I dropped by his store, and there he was standing cheerfully behind the counter hard at work. Surgery puts a great strain on your body and most patients feel tired. I recommend they remain active, but I also suggest they take frequent short rest periods. This was not an option for my clothing-store owner during the holiday season. But the lack of rest didn't seem to be doing him any harm.

His return to work was in striking contrast to another man recovering from simple disc surgery. Although his pre-operative leg pain had been cured, his general level of discomfort, recurrent nausea, and overwhelming fatigue made it impossible for him to go home. When I saw him on my daily rounds the next morning, I found him surrounded by family, several of whom were kneeling at the bedside. He was lying on the bed with his hands folded over his chest in funeral repose. The corner of the room was filled with flowers and cards. Everyone must have thought that major surgery required a major response. The family was amazed and, I suspect, appalled when I promptly discharged him. He left with his entourage of mourners in tow and spent the next three months playing out his role as the critically disabled convalescent.

### What about my long-term recovery?

Long-term recovery after a simple discectomy in the neck or low back is excellent. You should be able to return to all your normal activities with no permanent restrictions. Although your back is no longer normal (it has a scar on it), there is no reason for you to deny yourself any activity you wish. I strongly recommend you get into an exercise program and stay in shape. Having been through one operation is a great motivator to avoid another, if possible.

A number of factors can affect your recovery, just as a number of things can influence your neck and back pain. One of the most significant is your workers' compensation status. For reasons that are not entirely understood but are absolutely invariable, the success rate for spine surgery on compensation patients is about half of what you would expect in a non-compensation case. It is a fact of spine surgery that every compensation recipient should know before they agree to an operation.

### Is the problem likely to return?

The statistics suggest that another rupture of the same disc on the same side will occur in about one patient in ten, regardless of whether or not the interior of the disc is cleaned out. It is important to separate a true recurrence from a continuation of the original problem. A successful operation for acute sciatica should produce a minimum of six months, and preferably one year, of complete pain relief. After that time, any attack can be considered a new event. You should be treated as if the first operation had never taken place.

Because this type of surgery is quite limited, judging success is relatively easy. Patients who gain only a few weeks of pain relief before experiencing a return of back and leg pain are more likely to have had an unsuccessful operation than a recurrence. Patients whose pain remains unchanged after the surgery and only begins to improve six months or so later are more likely experiencing a spontaneous improvement than any delayed benefit of the surgery itself. Decompression surgery works right away. Recovery can continue for months but it should start within hours.

**You said there was no urgency about the operation except for my ability to withstand the pain. Can all back surgery be approached so slowly?**

Surgery for major trauma with a partial loss of spinal-cord function is performed urgently. So is some surgery for advancing spinal cancer where nerve function is being progressively lost.

The one absolute indication for urgent spine surgery in mechanical low back pain is a condition called acute cauda equina syndrome. (Remember, the cauda equina refers to the horse's tail of nerves in the spinal canal below the spinal cord.) Normally, a bulging disc irritates a single nerve within the bundle. Rarely, an extremely large rupture involving the entire back surface of the disc can quickly fill the canal and compress the entire tail. That can produce a sudden inability to urinate followed many hours later by an insensible and uncontrollable dribbling as urine collects in the bladder. There may be a loss of voluntary bowel control.

In this situation, decompression is an emergency. Statistics suggest that a delay of more than two days before removing the pressure on the nerves increases the risk that the patient will have permanent bowel and bladder dysfunction.

Acute cauda equina syndrome is extremely rare. It affects between 1 in 25,000 to 1 in 50,000 patients suffering an acute nerve-root compression. And nerve-root compression is the problem in only 10 per cent of the total back-pain population.

### If I have surgery on one disc, what is to prevent another disc from rupturing later on?

Nothing. If it does, it's just bad luck. But the statistics show that most back and neck pain is mechanical. Few people actually experience a pinched nerve. Even in that small group, most get better without surgery. Just because you had an operation for your first herniated disc doesn't mean you will need one for your second.

One patient of mine has gone through three operations for an acute herniated disc with nerve-root irritation. Two were at the same level and on the same side and the third was at the level below. The operations took place about two years apart, each time near Labour Day. The timing and the regularity of her surgery became a bit of an unhappy joke between us. But every operation was justified for a new problem, and all of them succeeded. In each instance, she had fully recovered and remained symptom-free for over a year. This patient simply had the rare misfortune of developing three separate disc herniations on three separate occasions. As luck would have it, I saw her on the street around Labour Day some years after her last successful surgery. We both agreed that this was a far better way to meet.

### So far you have mentioned decompression for disc ruptures and sciatica. What about surgery for Pattern 4?

Pattern 4, neurogenic claudication, can be caused by the reduced blood supply to the nerves as they crowd together within a small bony canal. Enlarging the canal is the surgical solution. Because the disc is not directly involved, it can be left untouched. The entire roof of the canal can be removed, a total laminectomy, or the individual constricted areas can be decompressed through a series of separate holes. These holes are called fenestrations, from the Latin word for window (they could also be called laminotomies or partial laminectomies). Both approaches appear to work, and the choice is largely a matter of the surgeon's preference.

### Is the success rate as good as for disc surgery?

Not always. If the narrow area is limited, the approach can be limited. Your stay in hospital will be similar to that for a simple disc procedure. But when the required decompression is more extensive, so is the size of the incision. That means more bruised muscle and a slower recovery.

Because decompression of a narrow canal is often performed in older patients, and because the spine keeps on ageing after the operation, the success of surgery for neurogenic claudication diminishes over time. Up to four patients in ten may return with a significant recurrence of their problem. Further decompression is possible, but the best course may be to return to an aggressive non-surgical approach for Pattern 4.

A narrow spinal canal in the neck compressing the spinal cord can present a surgical challenge. In these cases, the decompression may have to be carried out from both the back and the front. An extensive fusion to restore stability is almost always required.

## So a decompression is not always limited to a single level?

No, it is not. In most cases when a disc ruptures, only that disc needs to be decompressed. With canal narrowing, the length of the decompression depends upon the extent of the problem. For tumours and trauma, the surgery can involve one or many segments. In extreme cases, the decompression may require removing one or more complete vertebral bodies and the intervening discs. This is the only time a disc may be truly removed. The space is filled with a large bone graft, usually a portion of a leg bone obtained from the bone bank, and secured with a long plate and screws.

One other area where the excision usually extends over more than one level is in the coccyx, or tailbone. Pain in the area of the coccyx is called coccydynia (it is sometimes called coccygodynia; the terminology keeps getting in the way). Coccydynia describes the symptom of pain ("dynia" means pain) low down in the mid-line of the back. The name, no matter how it is spelled, says nothing about the cause of the problem. The tailbone can fracture with a fall on the backside or when giving birth. It may fail to unite properly and this can lead to years of local pain between the buttocks and great difficulty with sitting. Occasionally, removing several segments of the tailbone, a procedure called a coccygectomy, can resolve the symptoms. This operation should be approached with great caution. Pain in the coccygeal area frequently occurs when there is nothing wrong with the tailbone itself.

Pattern 1 and 2 low back pain is often felt in this location, and the pain in Pattern 1 typically worsens with sitting. Removing the coccyx in these cases won't solve the problem; it will probably make the situation worse.

### I saw something on television about using a laser to remove a disc. Do the new surgical techniques make a difference?

Whatever technique the surgeon selects, it should not decrease his success rate. The traditional open decompression and discotomy are the benchmarks against which the newer techniques must be compared.

Using magnifying loupes and a headlight or an operating microscope improves illumination and visibility. A decompression can be performed through a large tube pushed through the muscle, to minimize bruising, or with a video-assisted endoscope. The actual surgery can be performed with a scalpel or a cutting laser. The end result, removal of the offending structure, is the same.

The immediate goal is to minimize the invasiveness of the procedure, thereby reducing the post-operative pain and hastening recovery. But the ultimate goal remains an adequate decompression and a permanent resolution of the pre-operative problem. As impressive as some of the minimally invasive techniques appear, they do not always produce the same rate of success as the traditional methods. All of them take time to master, even for an experienced spine surgeon. Most of them limit the exposure and increase the risk of missing part of the problem. I am sure these approaches will continue to improve, but so will the routine operative procedures. The surgeon's decision to use a revolutionary new technique may have more to do with marketing and an ambition to be the first than with an analysis of the anticipated success and potential risks.

One rapidly evolving technical advance is computer-assisted surgery. After the spine is surgically exposed, a special probe locates specific anatomical landmarks and relays their locations by infrared or radio frequency signals to a computer. By combining these registration points with a pre-operative CT scan or a fluoroscopic image, the computer can produce a real-time three-dimensional X-ray of the spine during the operation. The program can precisely identify and measure specific structures and guide the placement of a screw. It can project the course of a drill before it is advanced. Such incredibly accurate images may not be necessary for a routine discectomy, but if the surgeon needs them, in a complex-deformity case or when fixing a fracture through the peg on top of C2, for example, they are available.

### Is there any way I can have a decompression but avoid surgery?

All the currently available procedures are invasive, meaning they break the skin. There are a few non-surgical options, but none of them delivers the same chance of success.

One alternative for treating the nerve irritation caused by an acute bulging disc is an injection that changes the disc's chemical structure. The procedure is called chemonucleolysis, and it uses a material derived from the papaya fruit, a substance similar to the tenderizer you use on a tough steak. The drug, chymopapain, does not dissolve the disc. It softens the disc by decreasing the molecular size and the bonding of proteins within the central nucleus. Figuratively speaking, it is like turning a walnut into a marshmallow. Since there is little change in the shape of the bulge, this alteration usually cannot be detected on a CT scan.

The procedure was first reported in the early sixties and over the years has maintained about a 70-per-cent success rate. It is safer than surgery. But it does have its own risks and complications. Chemonucleolysis can cause temporary acute back pain and severe muscle spasm. Very rarely, it can cause an extreme allergic reaction.

Chymopapain has lost much of its popularity. This may be due, in part, to the fact that although it is safer than surgery, its success rate is lower. I think a bigger reason it is no longer in vogue is the fact that it was frequently used to treat simple back-dominant pain. Chemonucleolysis may substitute for a decompression but it is not a treatment for back pain. Using any treatment for the wrong indications will guarantee its failure. A great number of patients were injected with chymopapain for back problems where the drug could not possibly have helped. As a result, its reputation was tarnished.

The indications for the use of chymopapain are slightly stricter than for a surgical decompression. If the injection fails to relieve acute sciatica, it should be followed by a conventional operation.

The controversy that surrounded chemonucleolysis is beginning to form around another minimally invasive technique for dealing with mechanical back pain. The new procedure is called interdiscal electro-thermal therapy (IDET). This time, the needle in the disc guides a fine heating filament that curls around the nucleus. The theory is that controlled levels of heat will contract and thicken the fibres of the disc wall, closing any small tears. The contraction can reduce the size of a disc bulge and the heat may also desensitize the nerves in the outer layers of the disc, its pain-sensitive region.

Like chymopapain, IDET is meant to alter the structure of the disc, but unlike chymopapain, IDET is intended to deal directly with discogenic pain. It is prescribed for patients with Pattern 1 symptoms.

Like so many new procedures, IDET was hailed as a major advance when it first appeared a few years ago. The initial reports were impressive. As time has passed, however, the percentage of excellent results seems to be falling, and two recent studies have put the level of improvement as about the same you might expect from a placebo. What is also disturbing is the fact that the patient's maximum improvement does not seem to occur until a year after the treatment. It is difficult to understand how any change in the disc structure would require so much time to have an affect. It may be significant that during the year after the procedure, patients are instructed to maintain an intensive supervised series of back-strengthening exercises.

Both chymopapain and IDET may have their place, but neither is the magic answer. I understand their appeal. A needle in your disc sounds a lot better than a knife in your back.

### It certainly does. Are there other treatments?

Yes, there are. One, called rhizotomy or rhizolysis, uses a needle to deliver a chemical, a high-energy radio pulse, or extreme cold to destroy the nerves that supply the small interlocking facet joints of the spine. Unlike the temporary anaesthetic block used to diagnose pain in these joints, rhizotomy intends to stop back pain permanently by destroying joint sensation. The procedure originally used a long knife. That was shown not to work. The current needle techniques have never been proven to be much better. Because the joints have more than one nerve supply, it is difficult to destroy them all. And when the body recognizes the injury, it attempts to repair it. Over time, some of the small joints recover their sensation and, presumably, their pain. Rhizotomy is another one of those procedures whose success rate can almost be accounted for by placebo effect.

Injecting minute amounts of a purified botulinum neurotoxin to temporarily paralyse the muscles of the face has become a very popular cosmetic procedure for relaxing wrinkles and age lines. The same material has received limited approval for the treatment of a rare neuromuscular disease that causes recurrent uncontrollable spasms in the neck and shoulder muscles. A few doctors have started offering injections of type-A botulinum toxin as a treatment for the muscle cramps that accompany mechanical neck and back problems. Since long-term pain control relies in part on increasing muscle strength along the spine, paralysing the same muscles for short-term pain relief seems to make little sense. At present, I believe this experimental use of a potentially dangerous compound should be avoided.

A different needle solution is called prolotherapy. It involves a series of shots to tighten up the ligaments of the spine or pelvis. Injections include high concentrations of sugar, salt, and phenol (carbolic acid). The theory is that these irritants will cause acute local inflammation resulting in scar tissue and increased stiffness. But inflammation does not always produce stiffness. In rheumatoid arthritis, for example, inflammation actually loosens the joints and allows them to separate. But even if the theory is correct, there is no evidence that back pain is regularly caused by loose joints. The whole idea is highly questionable. The technique is described in a few orthopaedic textbooks. But a careful review of the literature gives a very mixed picture. There can be serious complications with the injection of these noxious substances. The majority of spine experts do not believe prolotherapy is an acceptable treatment.

**Is that because prolotherapy is dangerous?**

In my opinion, it's because it's just a placebo. Doctors have underestimated the power of the patient's belief in the benefit of a particular treatment. Two recent publications having to do with knee surgery, not spine surgery, make this point very strongly. Both studies compared the conventional operation of cleaning and irrigating the painful arthritic knee with sham surgery. Patients in the sham group had the skin over their knee cut and sewed up but nothing whatsoever was done inside the joint. The result? The patients with sham surgery had a higher rate of success. Don't ever underestimate the power of placebo. And in a condition like back pain, where so many people get better without treatment or require nothing more than education and exercise, the placebo value of any invasive treatment with a knife or a needle is almost impossible to determine.

The situation is even more difficult and destructive when inappropriate surgery is performed on a pain-focused patient. The placebo effect often provides a short period of improvement that is inevitably followed by a complete relapse with even more pain and disability than before the operation. But now the patient can recount a miserable surgical experience and display a scar: visible proof of the severity of the physical problem and a permanent validation of the continuing invalid behaviour.

**So is there a placebo effect with spinal fusion?**

Probably. But there are circumstances in which fusing segments of the spine together may be the proper thing to do.

**When would you do a spinal fusion?**

Some of the indications are quite clear. A fusion is necessary if there has been a major spinal injury producing unstable fractures and dislocations. Even without nerve injury, a fusion may be necessary to realign the spine and permit healing in a normal position. Some malignant tumours of the spine may destroy enough bone to create instability, and a spinal fusion is the only means of solving that problem. After an extensive decompression of a narrow canal for Pattern 4 symptoms, the spine may be left without adequate stability and require a fusion. The only way to correct scoliosis surgically is to fuse the spine in its new position after it has been straightened. These types of fusions can extend over many levels.

Decompression through the front of the neck to relieve nerve pressure from a bulging disc in Pattern 3 removes a large amount of disc material. The space created between the vertebrae is usually filled with a block of bone. This fusion is required as a result of the decompression surgery.

The debate begins when spinal fusion is used to treat mechanical back and neck pain with no nerve-root irritation. Here, the surgeon usually fuses only one or two motion segments in an attempt to eliminate painful movement. Fusing for neck-dominant pain in the absence of Pattern 3 is unlikely to relieve the symptoms. Lumbar fusion doesn't always work for patients with typical Pattern 1 or Pattern 2 low-back symptoms either, but, flawed as it is, it may be the only thing we have to offer when adequate non-operative care fails.

### Are there a lot of risks?
The risks are the same as for a spinal decompression, but there are a few extra ones. Because the operation usually involves more muscle dissection and generally takes longer, the risks of infection and venous problems are greater. When the surgeon inserts hardware there is increased possibility that something will damage a nerve or the spinal cord. Some approaches can injure the large blood vessels that lead to and from the heart, or the collection of nerves at the back of the pelvis that control elements of sexual function in men. Complications are still very uncommon, but they are real, and they need to be considered and discussed.

### How do you fuse a spine?
Fusing the spine means convincing the body to grow bone bridges from one vertebra to the next. I sometimes suspect that with all the modern methods available, that basic point gets overlooked. The fusion doesn't depend on how strong the metal plate may be or how much wire the surgeon uses. It depends on getting the body to grow those bridges of bone.

Take the wire from a metal coat hanger and bend it. It seems strong enough. Now bend it in the opposite direction. Things still look good. Now bend it back and forth a hundred thousand times. I'll wait. Eventually, the metal will fatigue and break. The concept of metal fatigue is something we all understand. The metals used in a spinal fusion are stainless steel or titanium alloy, and they are far stronger than the metal in the coat hanger. But if they are bent repeatedly, they too will break.

But bone won't. Once the bridge is formed, the body will keep repairing and replenishing it. That section of your spine will be no different than the bone in your upper arm or lower leg. Once they are established, fusions never fail. Even a major spine injury will fracture the adjacent moving segments before it will break the fusion.

### Then why are so many people told that their fusion has failed?

The failure is not in the fused bone. The failure is in getting the fusion to take hold in the first place. Although the surgeon can prepare the way and offer strong encouragement, it is your own body that makes the fusion.

The basic principle is easy to understand. A bone's natural response to injury is to lay down more bone. If you break your arm, it heals by creating a cuff of new bone on either side of the fracture. The cuffs enlarge until they meet over the fracture and form a solid link. With time, new bone is strengthened and remodelled. Eventually, the broken bone regains its former shape.

I try to create the same environment in the spine. I strip off the muscles and ligaments that cover the bones. I remove a covering membrane, the periosteum, and then use a small power drill to score the surface lightly. I am sending a message to the vertebra that it has been fractured. To help the healing process, I take bone from a nearby part of the pelvis, cut it into small strips, or grind it up and carefully lay it from one vertebra to the next. This provides a scaffold over which the body can build its own cuff of bone. This new material also contains living cells with the potential of making more bone. I am not just relying on the vertebrae; I have brought up the reserves as well. In addition to damaging the surface of the vertebrae, I also open and destroy the small joints. By removing their smooth cartilage surfaces, I expose the raw underlying bone and leave a narrow gap that looks very much like a fracture. I pack that gap with bone.

Occasionally, when there is not enough of the patient's own bone, I can use specially treated human bone from a bone bank. Other options include prepared animal bone or artificial bone substitutes. There are several synthetic products available. They offer either the scaffold effect or bone growth stimulation. A few claim to do both.

Natural healing will begin within a few weeks. First, there will be bridges of fibrous tissue, and then bands of cartilage that join the vertebrae together. In a month or two, tendrils of bone will begin to cross the gap and, if all goes as planned, the fusion will begin. A solid link won't be established for five or six months, and the process of maturing or remodelling will continue for the next year or two. But once it is complete, the fusion is a living bridge that cannot fatigue as metal does. It will never fail.

### Are there any things I can do to help my back fuse?

Yes, there are. First, if you smoke, stop. Smoking has been clearly shown to interfere with the process of spinal fusion. There should be no smoking for at least six weeks before the surgery and six to twelve months afterwards.

Second, you can remain active. Bones respond favourably to use, just as muscles get bigger when you exercise. I am not talking about going out to pave your driveway, but I do want you walking and moving around. I recommend a light gym workout after the first month or so, starting with aerobic routines and moving carefully into a full fitness program.

### What about drinking more milk or taking vitamins?

Staying well-nourished is important. But unless you have a major deficiency, adding more vitamins and minerals won't help. The healing process proceeds pretty much on its own.

### So why do you need hardware?

In cases of trauma, tumour, or deformity, instrumentation is typically required to maintain the desired final position. In any fusion keeping both sides very still assists bone healing. It is not absolutely necessary (ribs heal while you keep breathing), but it is quite helpful. Because I am doing everything I can to coax the spine to fuse, I add metal to hold the bones rigidly in place. It is the same idea as using a clamp to hold two pieces of wood together while the glue dries. Once the glue has set, you don't need the vise any more.

Using hardware has become very popular in recent years. Although internal fixation has been available for decades, the newer designs and techniques have convinced many spine surgeons that they must use metal. The literature on the subject is not quite so definite. Bony fusion does occur without adding a fixation device. In some situations, the success rate doesn't seem to have changed at all in spite of the extra technical demands and expense. But if a fusion fails to develop, someone (and it may be the patient's lawyer) will want to know why the surgeon didn't use the most up-to-date techniques. There is a lot of pressure to stay current. Since both theory and practice suggest that hardware sometimes improves the result, why not use it?

Placing the screws in the vertebrae can be tricky. Usually they run down each side of the spinal canal through small columns of bone called the pedicles. If I am not doing a decompression, the canal remains closed and the position of the screws must be determined by the local anatomy and the feel of insertion, confirmed by fluoroscopy or an intraoperative X-ray.

The post-operative X-rays are dramatic, with all those large screws, bolts, and rods. That is what everyone sees, and that is usually what the surgeon talks about. The really important things on the X-ray are the little white wisps of bone that you can see lying alongside the spine. That is the fusion.

### If you don't need the hardware after the fusion, why not take it out?

After two years you can. But getting the metal out can be very difficult. If the fusion has laid down a lot of bone, some of that bone will grow over the hardware like a tree grows over a nail that was pounded into the bark years ago. Finding the hardware may mean cutting away the bone, and that doesn't make sense. The metal is completely inert and the body makes no attempt to reject it. If there is a particular reason why the hardware should be extracted, it can certainly be done.

## So, if you do everything right, you get a fusion?

I wish that were true. We don't understand enough about the fusion process to guarantee success. Careful technique and attention to the elements that promote bony union help, but even in the best of circumstances, a fusion is not guaranteed. Different surgeons give different statistics, yet even if I estimate a success rate of 80 or 90 per cent, that is no consolation to the patient whose fusion didn't take.

It gets even more complicated. The purpose of the fusion was to eliminate mechanical spine pain by eliminating painful movement and thus restore the patient to normal function. Unfortunately, even with a solid fusion, the pain does not always disappear. The effect can be devastating. Whether they will admit it to their surgeon or not, most patients dream of gaining a pain-free spine and a level of function they haven't enjoyed for twenty years. When that fails to happen, disappointment, depression, and growing hostility are fertile soil for the seeds of pain-focused behaviour.

Then there are patients in whom the fusion is clearly not secure, yet their pain has decreased and their function has improved. On the X-ray, no bone has formed, a rod has broken, or a screw has worked loose. But they feel better. That isn't the usual result, but it happens just often enough to keep us wondering if fusion is a placebo.

## How can you tell if the fusion is solid?

Not easily. A plain X-ray offers little help, and even the CT scan can be difficult to interpret. Taking X-rays with the patient bending as far forward and as far backward as possible can help. It should detect movement at the unfused levels and complete immobility at the site of the surgery. Adding hardware has actually made the identification of a failed fusion easier on the plain views. Without a solid bony union, any metal implant will eventually fail. The X-ray picture of broken fixation suggests that movement has continued. There is an interesting side effect of that failure. Improperly inserted hardware can actually hold the bones apart and retard the formation of the bone bridge. Once the metal gives way, the bones are free to move together and fusion may proceed as nature intended.

Hardware may help the assessment of a solid fusion on the plain X-rays, but it makes the interpretation more difficult with the CT. The X-ray beam scatters off the metal. The resulting interference can make it impossible to see the bone. Newer X-ray techniques and the use of titanium alloy implants that do not scatter the beam are helping to overcome the problem. In this case, CT is certainly a more sensitive investigation than plain X-ray. MRI does not do well with dry bone. It rarely adds useful information.

The X-ray or CT should show a continuous band of bone from one vertebra to another running at the back alongside the joints or forming between the bodies of the vertebrae. The location of the bone depends upon the site of the surgery. It is encouraging to see a loss of space within the spinal joints. When that gap is gone, the joint is presumably incapable of movement.

Some surgeons believe that the only way to be sure that a fusion has succeeded is to look at it directly. Even then, it can be difficult to be sure. The amount of remaining movement may be extremely small. It can occur in a direction other than the one the surgeon can see. The best indication of a solid fusion is probably a good clinical result, but even that is not certain.

### You haven't mentioned cages. Do they give a better fusion?

A "better" fusion is one with stronger bone between the vertebrae. A colleague of mine is fond of saying, "There are many ways to skin a cat but a cat without skin is still a skinned cat." Whether you achieve it with screws or rods or cages, or use no metal at all, a good fusion is a solid fusion.

Cages come in various shapes and sizes. Their supposed advantage is that they are placed in the front of the spine between the flat surfaces of the vertebral bodies. The cages are hollow and filled with the patient's bone obtained from the pelvis or from the backs of the vertebrae. They are usually inserted in pairs between the vertebrae to be fused and the remaining space around them is packed with more bone. It is still the bone that makes the fusion.

Using cages brings up another aspect of technique: fusing the spine from the front rather than from behind, as I have already described. Cages are commonly inserted from the front, as are the bone blocks typically used in cervical fusion. Fusing from the front and implanting cages in the low back means going through the abdomen or slipping around the side of the abdominal cavity. The skin incision is at the front and there is no scar on your back. If the cages are judged to provide sufficient support, there is no need to disrupt the spinal muscles. However, many surgeons doubt the stability of anterior standalone cages, particularly when more than one level is being fused, and always supplement them with posterior hardware inserted through a separate incision in the back.

Cages can also be placed from behind. Inserting a cage through the spinal canal requires cutting a large hole in the lamina, moving the nerves a considerable distance out of the way and adding additional instrumentation. Because putting in a cage posteriorly requires so much space and retraction of the nerves, it is not a suitable operation for the neck. The cervical spinal cord hates to be disturbed. Posterior fusions in the cervical spine use only rods or plates secured with screws.

Fusing between the vertebral bodies allows more area for contact. The more surface contact, the more space your body has to build those bone bridges. Fusing at the front of the spine also takes advantage of the fact that, for much of the time, the vertebral bodies are subjected to load while the joints at the back are under tension. A graft at the front is squeezed together and held rigidly. A graft at the back is more prone to movement and may be pulled slightly apart.

Operating from the front has a final advantage: it does not disturb the muscles along the spine. Damaging those muscles when you fuse the spine from behind seems to defeat part of your purpose, which is to enable the patient to resume normal activity and exercise rapidly.

In spite of the theoretical advantages, fusing from the front has not been shown to produce a significantly better clinical result. Your chance of eliminating mechanical back or neck pain with a spinal fusion seems to be about the same whether you approach the spine anteriorly or posteriorly.

### What can I expect after a spinal fusion?
Your stay in hospital will be similar to that for a spinal decompression, but you are unlikely to go home the same day or the next morning. Thirty or

forty years ago, patients undergoing spinal fusion were kept in hospital for months and maintained on a special turning frame or rotating bed. Today, because of the stability provided by the instrumentation, most fusion patients are allowed out of bed the next morning and will go home within a few days. If the surgery is done from behind, the incision is longer than for most decompressions. More muscle is bruised, so initially the back hurts more. If surgery is done from the front, patients usually have very little back pain and their early mobilization is easier.

In the neck, when the fusion is done from the front we often use a small plate. The hardware used with the posterior approach is the same as that used in the low back, only smaller. For the first month or so, cervical fusions are generally protected part of the time with a collar. With the new hardware, most short low-back fusions do not require a brace at all.

I am quite aggressive with post-fusion rehabilitation. You will not compromise the success of the fusion by being active or returning to a supervised exercise program. I remember one patient whom I met while he was exercising in a CBI clinic. In spite of his best efforts (he was a non-smoker and well-nourished), his fusion failed to consolidate. His surgeon blamed the clinic for allowing his patient to be active. The exercise program under attack consisted of a light treadmill routine, some time on an exercise bicycle, and a little bench work with light weights. None of it put undue stress on the spine and it was not responsible for the failure to fuse. I guess the surgeon didn't want to be accused of poor surgical technique. Sometimes fusions just don't happen.

## What are the long-term results of spinal fusion?

The loss of movement at one or more levels in the spine puts an extra strain on the adjacent discs and joints. The junction between the moving parts and the immobile section can be the site of future trouble. Half of all patients who undergo spinal fusions will develop problems in this area. Several things can happen. The most obvious is an accelerated wear on the neighbouring disc. Although this is common, it rarely produces enough trouble to justify extending the fusion. Narrowing of the spinal canal can occur as well, but the amount of pressure on the nerves is seldom sufficient to warrant decompression.

Surgeons have come to recognize the importance of re-establishing the normal spinal curves. Failure to maintain the proper lordosis in the neck or low back can lead to a loss of spinal balance and leave the post-fusion patient unable to stand properly upright. In the neck, this leads to persistent pain. In the low back, it produces a condition called flat-back syndrome. The loss of proper spinal alignment causes low back pain and requires the patient to rely heavily on the leg muscles to stand straight. That results in leg pain and fatigue. In both areas, the loss of correct spinal balance is believed to contribute to accelerated degeneration of the adjacent levels.

Most people and many surgeons do not realize that almost half of the normal curve in your low back occurs within the lowest two segments. Since these are also the most commonly fused levels, maintaining the lordosis when the bones are positioned for fusion is critical.

### If you don't get a fusion the first time, can you try again?

Yes, but the probability of success is dramatically reduced. Unless the initial surgical technique was very poor, whatever prevented the fusion from happening the first time is likely to interfere again. Cleaning the spine is more difficult through the scar tissue from the first procedure. Locating the anatomical landmarks for accurate placement of the hardware can be almost impossible. Because the bone has already been damaged, you have to do even more to convince the body to start to fuse.

When a second fusion is to be done, it is often wise to change the direction from which you approach the spine. If the first attempt was from behind, then the second might be done best from the front. Sometimes the second surgery should be from the front and back, a "360-degree fusion." Fusing from both directions is like holding up your pants with your belt and your suspenders; you try everything you can. It increases the amount of surgery, but it may help.

With spinal fusions, your first chance is your best chance and your second chance may be your last. The probability of success for a third procedure is about 30 per cent. The chance of succeeding decreases with each subsequent attempt. Multiple surgeries also increase the risk of serious complications. There is a far greater probability of nerve injury, major vessel damage, or infection than with the first operation. The surgeon has a greater likelihood of making the patient worse than of making him or her better. And even if there are no operative mishaps, the psychological effects of multiple failed operations are overwhelming. Pain-focused behaviour is certain, and further treatment, operative or otherwise, may be impossible. Some surgeons use surgically implanted morphine pumps in the spinal canal or electrical stimulators inserted next to the spinal cord. None of these salvage procedures works very well. None provides complete pain relief. It is a sad comment on the number of people whose spine surgery is unsuccessful that their situation has been accorded its own name: failed back-surgery syndrome.

Here is a regrettably typical story. A sixty-year-old man was diagnosed with a severe case of canal narrowing, producing Pattern 4 leg pain from neurogenic claudication. An extensive decompression eliminated his symptoms. Three years later, he was involved in a minor car accident and his symptoms returned with a vengeance. At the second surgery, there was a thick ridge of scar tissue running across the area of the previous decompression. The accident had either added more scar or disrupted a delicate balance between the amount of scar in his spine and the pressure on the local nerves. Removing the scar and enlarging the canal gave a second satisfactory result.

A year later, his back pain recurred. A third operation to further enlarge the canal revealed a mass of scar tissue strangling the nerve sac. Surgery to remove scar only causes more scarring and is never successful. In this case, further enlargement of the canal required removal of the remnants of several of the interlocking joints. It produced obvious instability. The fourth operation was a spinal fusion. Four operations left the patient with pain-focused behaviour, significant mechanical restrictions to normal back function, and leg pain brought on by walking: the same leg pain that had prompted the first surgery.

## Are there any treatments I can have instead of fusion?

Destroying the nerves to the facet joints and heating the interior of the disc are two of the options. Neither produces a particularly good result.

One less invasive option shows promise for limited indications. First used in Europe in the mid-1980s, it was designed to manage the painful compression fractures that occur with osteoporosis. Its minimally invasive nature is advantageous because the compression fractures are typically found in older people, who might not withstand major spinal surgery. The procedure is called vertebroplasty.

Under X-ray control, a large-bore needle is inserted through the pedicle of the vertebra into the collapsed vertebral body. Bone cement, the same kind used in hip-replacement surgery, is injected through the needle and into the fracture space. The cement stabilizes the bone immediately. For the small number of people for whom a compression fracture remains painful, this procedure can seem miraculous. The excruciating back pain is gone the moment the patient leaves the X-ray table.

A variation of vertebroplasty is called kyphoplasty. A large-bore needle is used to introduce a heavy balloon into the vertebral body. The balloon is inflated and opens up a space inside the broken bone. If done early, it can restore much of the vertebral height. That is something that vertebroplasty cannot do. Once the space is created, the balloon is removed and the bone cement is injected. Since both procedures are relatively new, neither approach has yet been shown to be superior over the other. Both have their benefits and their drawbacks, but in one form or another, this minimally invasive solution will be around for some time.

As with most spine surgery, kyphoplasty has complications. The cement can be accidentally pushed into the spinal canal or flow into a blood vessel. As the number of cases done grows and more time elapses after the cement insertion, new problems are appearing with the collapse of the fragile vertebrae beside the cement-filled one. No one yet knows how serious this complication will become.

Cement injection is now used with spinal metastatic tumours. In patients too weak to withstand major spine surgery, part of the tumour can be extracted through the needle and replaced with bone cement. The procedure reduces pain and improves stability. Because the adjacent bones are healthy, the problem of neighbouring vertebral collapse does not occur.

There have been other advances. Many centres are experimenting with artificial discs. It is hoped that the artificial disc will do for the spine what artificial hips and knees have done for the worn joints in your legs. Before major joints could be replaced, the only surgical way to stop severe arthritic pain was to fuse the joint so it could not move. Having your hip or knee fused in one position made many activities difficult and others impossible. Joint replacement revolutionized joint surgery, but the situation in the spine is not quite the same. Fusing a segment of the spine does not immobilize your back. With the exception of the first two levels of the neck below the skull, one motion segment contributes only a small amount to the overall movement. Patients with a single fused level can detect no change in their back movement. Many actually report improvement after fusion, since the remaining function is pain-free. Those who advocate the artificial disc point to the fact that, over time, levels adjacent to a fusion will wear out more rapidly. But that wearing-out can take twenty years or more. Artificial discs have not been around long enough to allow us to know if they will do any better. A successful disc replacement gives a result comparable to a successful fusion, but sometimes they don't even work that well. They have no place in spine surgery for trauma or tumours. It's still not clear that using an artificial disc instead of a fusion for back pain is the correct answer.

The problem is not an easy one, and many different solutions are being considered. Some artificial discs are mechanical: a metal and plastic combination like the ball-and-socket joint of the hip joint, only much flatter. Other researchers are attempting to replicate the action of the disc nucleus by inserting water-absorbing gelatins inside the disc's own shell. Artificial disc procedures have been carried out in both the neck and low back. They are highly experimental, and at this point no one knows which of the two techniques will be the most successful. Perhaps neither will work and an entirely new approach will take the day. So far, no one has attempted to replace both the disc and the corresponding spinal joints. The motion segment is proving to be far more complex than we had previously thought.

Bone mineral protein (BMP) obtained through genetic manipulation appears to have the potential to produce solid bony fusion in every patient without the need for any form of fixation. Perhaps someday it will simply be injected into the spine, eliminating the need for surgery. Future historians may consider surgery on the spine to relieve back and neck pain as primitive as trepanning holes in the skull to release evil spirits.

# CHAPTER THIRTEEN

## *Off to Work We Go*

Whether it is fair or not, the most commonly used measure of success following spine surgery or spine rehabilitation is the patient's ability to return to work. It may not seem as personally important as pain relief, or as objective as measuring the return of muscle power, but it is a widely accepted benchmark of recovery. Return to work serves as a proxy for return to normal activity. You can usually measure the first, but only estimate the second. Announcing that you have returned to your job is assumed to mean you have also fully resumed personal activities like gardening, wind surfing, or the bridge group.

To confound the issue further, the result being observed may not be return to work at all. Just as work is considered a proxy for activity, the termination of insurance benefits or the closing of a compensation claim may stand in for actually resuming employment. But in the analysis of success for the patient, they are not synonymous. Coverage may lapse and compensation be denied while the claimant is still physically or emotionally unable to return to the job.

A patient's ability or willingness to return to work depends upon many factors other than the health of his or her back or neck. The end result of successfully getting back to the job represents a string of variables that cannot be predicted or assessed.

A patient I recently saw illustrates how easily returning to regular work can differ from returning to normal activity. This man's problem was not something as potentially complicated as a back problem. He had fractured a bone in his foot. While at work, a slab of steel struck his boot just above the metal toe cap and broke a bone on the outside edge of his foot. It was obviously a painful injury and he couldn't keep working.

Fractures in the foot heal in the same fashion as broken bones everywhere else in the body. Because we constantly abuse our feet by walking miles every day, foot injuries tend to stay painful for quite a long time. His doctor asked me to see the patient three months after the injury because his foot still hurt and he had been unable to go back to work. I took new X-rays that showed excellent healing. Some early remodelling indicated the bone was rapidly returning to normal. As expected, it was still sore.

Because he had not worked for three months and was apprehensive about going back to his job, I recommended that the patient start on a part-time basis. That would ease the discomfort in his foot and gradually restore his confidence in his own ability. I assumed, wrongly, that my brief consultation would be my last contact with him.

His doctor asked me to see the same patient six months later. New X-rays showed such a degree of healing that it was almost impossible to locate the site of the fracture. Squeezing on his foot didn't hurt and he told me that he only felt pain at the end of a long day of standing and walking around. He was at work but still on the part-time schedule I had suggested as a temporary measure six months earlier. I asked him to walk on his tiptoes and then on his heels. I asked him to jump up and down. Nothing hurt. I asked what he was doing outside of the job. He told me he had returned to all of his normal activities and was having no trouble. So I asked why he was still only part-time. He told me that his doctor refused to permit him to resume a full-time schedule as long as his foot hurt at all. The patient's failure to return to his regular job had nothing to do with his rate of healing or his residual pain. It was the result of inappropriate restrictions applied by his family physician.

I recommended that he resume his job on a full-time basis immediately and provided him with the necessary medical authorization. It is impossible to know someone else's motivation, so I half expected him to tell me he agreed with his doctor and that he felt he was not capable of completing a full day's work. Instead, he said, "I was really counting on you telling me that. My boss said if I didn't come back full-time they were going to have to let me go."

His doctor's well-intentioned caution almost cost this patient his job. This case was just a simple foot fracture. You can see how much more difficult it would be to accept that mechanical neck and back pain don't need to be protected forever; to accept that the best thing to do, pain and all, may be to go to work.

### I am sure my insurance company/compensation board/employer wants me to go back to work just so they can stop paying benefits. Why should I go back so soon?

Most people don't realize that work can be therapeutic. We generally think of ourselves in terms of what we do. When you meet someone for the first time and ask him who he is, he will generally identify himself by telling you what he does.

"Hi, who are you?"

"I'm the new bank manager."

Without the security of work, many of us lose our identity and with it our sense of purpose and well-being.

"Hi, who are you?"

"I'm a chronically disabled neck-pain sufferer."

Work also adds structure to our lives. Whether you have a job or not, you live in a world of workdays and weekends. You share society's quiet despair of Monday morning and revel in Friday afternoon. Work puts a timetable in your day. It directs when you will wake in the morning and suggests when you should go to bed at night. One of the hallmarks of pain-focused behaviour is a loss of that structure. Days become numbingly similar, with nothing to break the monotony.

"What are you going to do today?"

"Probably what I did yesterday, which is pretty much what I did the day before, I think. What day is this, anyway?"

## But isn't working with a sore back/sore neck bad for me?

On the contrary, it will improve your rate of functional recovery. Having something to do provides purpose and motivation. Getting the job done requires increased activity and physical exertion. That's what your back or neck needs too.

Being at work may actually let you hurt less. It is a question of focus. Paying attention to the job leaves less time for you to be absorbed by your pain. And that is a good thing.

Dr. William Fordyce, an expert in pain management, said, "People don't hurt as much when they have something better to do."

## That's all well and good, but my neck/back injury is too serious for me to go back to work.

That may be. It is far more likely that going back to work won't cause you any harm at all. Hurt is not harm. But your expectations of hurt and harm can do a great deal of damage. When it comes to neck and back pain, most people have remarkably low expectations for their recovery. And those poor expectations can become self-fulfilling prophecies. If you believe you will fail, then fail you will.

Twenty years ago, I was part of a research group looking at treatment outcomes and comparing them to patients' self-reports of the severity of their own problems. We used a well-accepted, validated questionnaire to get that information. We had access to the clinical records, so we knew how serious each patient's medical condition really was. What we found was that a successful return to work depended more on what the patient believed would happen than on any medical parameters. It mattered less if someone was seriously injured than whether or not they believed they would recover. That belief appeared to be independent of the injury or the treatment.

## So why don't people expect to be normal again?

One reason is the widespread belief that neck and back pain are usually serious and mark the start of a lasting disability. That is not true, but the belief persists. And that misconception is supported by medical practice.

About ten years ago, our research group at CBI published the results of a study involving 1,400 patients. In the first half of the study, patients received the standard medical instructions when they were discharged from treatment: "If it hurts, don't do it. Your treatment has been successful, but you should still let pain be your guide." Doctors and therapists generally put a good deal of emphasis on pain. In this first group of patients, 44 per cent were told to return to their usual job in an unrestricted fashion. Thirty-seven per cent were instructed to go back to work, but only in some type of modified capacity.

For the second phase, we changed the rules. The participating clinicians were directed to permit job modification only when there was objective evidence of physical impairment. Pain alone would not be accepted as a legitimate reason to prescribe reduced activity. To make it even more unattractive for the treating professionals to limit the patient's return to work, the reasons for every restriction were to be submitted in writing to the research group. It is important to note that in the second group, there were no changes in the length or nature of the treatment. The analysis of the two groups showed no difference in the average age, ratio of men to women, nature of work, or severity of injury. The two groups were the same. But among the second sampling, 81 per cent of the patients had received a recommendation to return to work in an unrestricted fashion. Only 8 per cent had qualified for modified duty.

## But that just reflects the fact that you made it harder to restrict someone's return to work!

That's right, but that is not the point of the study. Two members of the research team contacted all 1,400 patients six months after discharge to find out whether they had complied with the recommendation they got at the end of their treatment. The two researchers found that in the first phase, when the advice to return to full duty was given 44 per cent of the time, 89 per cent of the patients complied. They went back to a regular routine and were working normally. In the second group, the recommendation to return to full duty was given 81 per cent of the time and 84 per cent of the patients still complied and were working in an unlimited fashion. The difference in the actual number of people working normally in each group is startling. Just telling people that they were able to do their job almost doubled the number who successfully returned to their regular work. We also found that instructing employees to return to work in a limited fashion statistically increased the chance that they would fail to go back to work at all.

### If the recommendation for limited duty is so harmful, why do doctors use it?

I don't think most doctors are aware of the potential damage. They are trying to help their patient become active again. Starting slowly seems to makes sense. What they don't see is the mixed message they are sending. To the patient they say, "You have made a full recovery." But when they insist that the patient's activities be limited, it's like they are saying, "Actually, you're not as well as I said you were, so you have to be careful." That same confusing message is heard by the employer, who may find it difficult to make the necessary accommodations, or who may decide that it would be easier to hire an able-bodied worker.

There are times when modified work makes sense. When someone has been away from the job for several months, climbing back into harness can be both physically and emotionally challenging. Imagine that you had not worked at your regular job for over a year. How would you feel on the first morning you returned? Going back for a few hours and then having the chance to rest might be an excellent idea. But the transition should be brief and finite, with a definite plan for the resumption of full duty.

If modification is recommended, it is better to adjust the time schedule than to modify the job. People returning from a back or neck injury are sometimes put into so-called light duties as a way of protecting them from further injury. In a misguided attempt to help, the employer may decide that instead of the usual job in the warehouse that required a combination of walking, standing, lifting, and climbing, the newly recovered worker should be started in the office, where he or she must sit all day. Sitting puts a greater load on the discs in the back than does standing or walking. There is a good chance that if the worker were given freedom to adjust the pace of the work and to get assistance for heavy lifting, the job in the warehouse would cause less back or neck pain than being trapped at a desk in the office.

Many of these transitional jobs are pointless tasks. It is hard to generate much enthusiasm for going back to a job like that. Several years ago, I worked with one company that had a much better answer. The managers set apart several segments of the assembly process where the work was not physically demanding or tightly time-constrained, and created a job re-entry area. Workers returning after back or neck injury started in this area with jobs they could manage and that were an essential part of the overall assembly. They were needed, and what they did was important. They were not supervised by someone from the health department but by their regular supervisor. They didn't look up to see the company nurse; they saw their old boss. The project was so successful that the demand for the re-entry positions grew rapidly and that brought a bonus. With so many applicants, the pressure to move workers through the "modified assembly area" insured that no one was left mouldering in a light-duty position.

Another reason doctors impose inappropriate job modifications is because of their attention to pain. Patients with neck and back trouble come to the doctor primarily so that the doctor can make the pain go away. Why would that same doctor do anything that might make the pain come back? In another project at CBI, we looked at the reasons that people gave for using rehabilitation after a spinal injury. We interviewed nearly six hundred patients. Some of the patients were already at work, others had been off the job for a long time. Some were receiving financial assistance for their treatment, others had to cover the cost themselves. Regardless of the circumstances, the first reason the patients gave for attending rehabilitation was pain control. We then interviewed over a hundred doctors who had referred their patients for therapy. Whether the individual was at work or not, the doctors' primary reason for the referral was pain control. The doctors were attempting to provide what their patients demanded. When our researchers interviewed the people who usually pay the bills for treatment (insurance companies and compensation boards), we found that if a claimant was off work, their principle intent was to get him or her back on the job. If the claimant was already working, their goal was to improve the claimant's function. Pain control, which was the principal concern of the patients and doctors, was not the overriding consideration for the payers. With such an obvious mismatch in the anticipated objectives of treatment, it is little wonder we see hostility develop between claimants, their doctors, and the paying agencies.

**But you say that the insurance company is right. Pain should not be a reason to stay off work.**

Pain is not a medical reason to restrict work, but it is an enormous disincentive. If your job requires you to perform a task that hurts every time you do it and your typical pain steadily increases through the day, you are not likely to enjoy your work. Recently, I spent some time cutting bush trails. I found the work enjoyable when I started, but after several hours with the chainsaw and a lot of heavy lifting, my back decided it had had enough. If that had been my job and my boss demanded that I report for duty again early the next morning, I doubt I could have made it. But I had done myself no harm. My back pain was not an indication of a problem requiring medical attention. My pain was not a basis for a medical restriction. I am not saying that pain can be ignored. There will be situations when pain makes certain tasks impossible. I am saying the decision not to work because of pain should be made by the sufferer, not the doctor. Physicians often tell me their role is to advocate for their patients. The true advocate promotes what is best for the client. I believe in most instances that what is best for the bad back or the sore neck is to keep going.

**So what should the doctor do?**

Make a recommendation rather than a restriction. This is not just word play. A restriction implies that any violation will lead to serious, possibly permanent consequences. You are restricted from climbing a high-tension electrical tower because the current could kill you. A recommendation offers the best option but leaves you with the freedom to make a choice. When your friend recommends that you pass on a movie that she thinks is stupid, you still have the option to go and see for yourself.

When doctors lay down unnecessary restrictions and impose limits that are often exceeded by their patients, two unwanted results occur. First, the patient is subjected to unnecessary fear: believing that by stepping out of bounds, they are risking permanent physical injury. Second, when they ignore the restrictions, they are unlikely to tell the doctor, and an opportunity to discuss better alternatives and strategies to work within the limits of the pain is lost.

### Then a well-meaning doctor may actually be a barrier to the patient's return to work?

The unnecessary restrictions certainly are. The assumed role of advocate can get in the way, as well. I remember talking to one doctor who was adamant that his patient with the sore neck should not be allowed to return to work as a welder on a government project. After several minutes I realized that none of the doctor's concerns were related to his patient's physical problems. The doctor's concerns and his advocacy centred on the fact that due to a recent downsizing, the government was forcing his patient to do a job formerly allotted to three men. He was being asked to put in longer hours and work faster then he had ever done before. It was the employment situation that angered the doctor. As I recall, we never did discuss the weight of the welding helmet, cervical discs, muscles, or biomechanics. Finally, the doctor announced to me, "I don't think it's fair that someone should have to work with pain." It may not be fair, and it certainly isn't pleasant, but it may be the only available option. It may also be the best thing for your neck.

### Are there any other barriers blocking a return to work, even if the doctor gives me permission?

There are several. Many, like the increased demands on the welder, have nothing to do with the medical situation. In a faltering economy, one of the largest barriers may be that there is simply no job available. There is nothing the doctor can do about that. But there are ways the physician can be of some assistance. Don't place restrictions that will narrow a job applicant's opportunities. Don't prescribe ineffective medical therapy. The emphasis should be on finding a job, not applying a TENS unit.

Return to work may be hampered by unrecognized conflicts. Problems may exist in the workplace, about which the doctor knows nothing. Injured workers can become involved in hostile confrontations with the compensation board or the disability carrier. The more the injured party feels pressured to return to work for reasons other than personal benefit, the more likely it is that the patient will present the doctor with a dramatic increase in the symptoms and a magnification of the disability. Without insight into the real problems, these physical symptoms may prompt the doctor to add restrictions and carry out further unnecessary medical treatments.

Not everyone who sustains a neck or back injury recovers completely. A small number are left with lasting physical limitations, like weakness in muscles controlled by a particular nerve. In these cases, permanent job modification may be necessary, and the availability of suitable employment can become another barrier. I have never seen a more dramatic representation of this problem than when I examined two patients, one after the other, in a workers' compensation clinic. The first patient was a man with chronic low back and neck pain. It did not take long for me to determine that his major problem was a well-established and unshakeable pattern of pain-focused behaviour. He was not working because no one could find him suitable employment: that special job that would not irritate any of his numerous aches and pains. The next patient on my list was a man who had been critically injured in a mining explosion. He had been a hard-rock miner and had no other job skills. The explosion had cost him both legs and one arm. And he was working. He had taken courses in mine safety and was employed as a safety supervisor and lecturer on safe mine practices. I suspect he could tell an enthralling story. I will never forget those two men, nor underestimate the importance of working to your full potential regardless of your physical handicap or level of pain.

**Are you saying the man with the back pain was more disabled than the man with the missing limbs?**

The concept of disability is not an easy one to understand. We often confuse disability with physical impairment, and they are not the same. The most frequently used example is that of a man who loses the tip of his fifth finger on his non-dominant hand. If he is a labourer, the loss of a small bit of an unimportant digit will not interfere with his job. It will produce no disability. If the man is a concert pianist, that small physical loss will translate into a substantial disability. Physical impairment is what the doctor can see and measure. But the degree of physical impairment does not dictate the level of disability. Determining disability requires knowledge of the work or activity that must be done and an assessment of how the physical impairment will adversely impact those tasks. When the problem is neck and back pain, a complaint so rarely linked with any objective physical findings, establishing levels of disability can be a daunting task. It is one reason why neck- and back-related injuries are such a contentious basis for workers' compensation claims or permanent disability appeals.

A colleague of mine, an occupational physician, makes a distinction between absolute disability and activity avoidance. If there is objective evidence of a total incompatibility between the observed physical impairment and the fully defined job requirements, determining an absolute disability is relatively straightforward. Prescribing activity avoidance is quite different. It requires a judgement by the physician that a patient's particular physical limitations will interfere with a specific set of activities. It is a judgement that is not always accurate. There are many ways of accomplishing the same task. Underestimating the patient's ingenuity or misinterpreting the demands of the activity may render the doctor's opinion invalid. Activity avoidance can also be self-imposed. Patients who fear their pain, or who have been led to believe that an activity is harmful, may elect not to attempt working and to withdraw themselves from the job market. This voluntary withdrawal, based on complaints of neck and back pain, may be erroneously and unfortunately supported by the worker's physician.

**So if there's too much pain, a worker may just choose not to work?**
Whether to work or not is a choice that we can all make. Many of us enjoy our jobs, but if you won the lottery, you might find other ways to spend your time. It is impossible to determine someone else's motivation. We can believe what people tell us, but we can't read their minds. Proof of a desire to work comes through action and that action is controlled by many things other than the physical condition of the spine.

In Chapter 10, I talked about the components of secondary gain: financial support, attention, control of your surroundings, and escape from an unpleasant situation. These all directly affect the decision to return to work and must be taken into account. Failing to consider these factors can lead the doctor to investigate and treat a condition unconnected to the real problem.

**What strategies do you suggest for getting someone back to work?**
Emphasize the benign nature of neck and back pain. Stress the self-limiting nature of every acute attack. Eliminating fear, particularly fear that work will harm the spine, is the best place to start. Provide enough anatomy education to ensure the patient understands that the spine is strong and stable, that discs don't slip, and that backs never go out. Most important of all, give the responsibility for recovery back to the patient. The injured party must take control, not wait for someone else to solve the problem.

Three workers in ten who suffer a neck or back injury will be on the job again within seventy-two hours and will not file a claim for lost time. They need support for that decision from their doctor, their family, and their friends. For those who must leave work, early and regular contact with the employer is important. Knowing that you are missed at work and that accommodations can be made for your return is reassuring. Initial treatment need be no more than basic education and pain-relieving modalities. The focus must be on early resumption of normal activities. Any delay can retard the rehabilitation process.

Allowing an injured worker to remain off work without a plan for recovery makes things worse. I recall one woman who told me she had not had contact with her employer at all since her accident eight months earlier. I suggested she get in touch, and that is how she learned the company had relocated out of town and her job had vanished. The sooner patients with back and neck injuries get involved in rehabilitation planning, the less likely it is that sort of breakdown in communication will occur.

There is the question of when it is safe for someone with a neck or back injury to return to work. In the absence of major trauma with a spinal fracture or a Pattern 3 with significant neurological impairment, the answer is usually right away. It may not be easy, but if it's possible, it should be arranged. The sooner an injured worker returns to the job, the better it will be for everyone concerned, most of all the injured worker.

One useful trick is to schedule the first day of work in the later half of the week. Going back to the job on Monday revives those old unpleasant feelings. Going back to work on Thursday means you're just one day from the weekend and the chance to relax. It may only be a mind game, but anything that eases the transition from weeks of pain-filled immobility to a busy day at the office or in the plant is worth trying.

The most successful rehabilitation outcome places an injured worker back in the old job with the old employer. When that is not possible, the next best option is for the worker to find different employment within the same company. When that too is beyond reach, the third option should be the original job in a new setting. Only as a last resort should the injured worker be cast completely adrift to begin a new occupation in a new workplace.

### That last option sounds frightening. Do people in that situation often succeed?

Not very often. I remember a woman whom I saw for a rehabilitation assessment. She had been away from her job as a municipal bus driver for two years because of continuing back pain. In that time, she had come to realize that there were other things she could do to earn a living. With the aid of the compensation board, she had gone back to school and begun training as a chartered accountant. It was hardly a choice I would have anticipated, but she was succeeding brilliantly. Her failure to return to work had created an opportunity that might never have existed had her early treatment been successful. I remember her because her story was so unusual and so far from the routinely disastrous results of delaying.

This is not a typical case, but it is an excellent example of what taking control can do. This woman's decision to go back to school was not something she was forced into by a vocational counsellor. It was a decision she took for herself after she had reviewed her options. It helped that she had the ability to match her drive. Not everyone who washes dishes in a diner can become president of the bank. Having realistic expectations is important. Many people claim they would like to take the opportunity offered by the injury to change their lives for the better. But that change takes hard work and an honest appraisal of their opportunities. As a doctor, I can help solve the physical problems. So much more depends upon the attitude of the injured worker.

## What can a doctor do to improve an injured worker's attitude?

Try to keep the situation simple. When simple conditions are treated in a complicated fashion, they become complicated. Patients become frightened and the easy steps to recovery become difficult. Explain the medical situation in understandable language and reinforce the positive aspects of the problem. Help the patient make the correct decision to work through the pain.

The doctor should encourage the worker to remain in touch with his or her employer and to stay tied emotionally and geographically to the workplace. Even if the injured worker can't do the job, contact can be maintained by stopping by the shop at lunch or coffee break. A sore back shouldn't stop the worker from maintaining workplace friendships. Being cut off from co-workers means being cut off from a large part of life. That may leave little to do but dwell on the pain and magnify the image of his or her disability.

The sooner the injured worker goes back to work, the better. There are few reasons to delay. The benefits of a prompt resumption of activities far outweigh the small risk of further injury.

One of the most important things is to coordinate all the recommendations and requirements that the injured worker receives. What the patient hears from the doctor should be the same as what is heard from the physio-therapist, the vocational counsellor, the insurance adjuster, and the employer. If patients receive mixed messages, they become confused or they select the message that best suits their personal agenda. If you do not want to go back to work but everyone insists that you must try, you will probably make an attempt. But when your therapist advocates exercise while your doctor counsels rest, you tend to choose the advice you want to hear. When your doctor recommends you return to work but your employer stipulates that you must be "100 per cent," you have a choice of going back to the job and proving you can do it, or going back to your doctor and complaining that your boss won't let you work. It is frustrating how seldom all the involved parties have the opportunity to discuss the situation and reach a common understanding. If their goals are not the same, how can they all hope to succeed? If they share the same objective, loopholes are closed, tech-nical failures are avoided, and the injured worker has only one path to follow: the path to recovery.

Perhaps there is no stronger force for or against the return to work than expectancy. People usually respond in the way they are expected to respond. And because the expectations for recovery after neck and back injury are so low, it is imperative to correct that mistaken belief. We all act as we are expected to act, just as we see what we expect to see: the numbers 1 and 3 placed closely together, and appearing between the letters A and C, become the letter B, not the number 13. The injured worker who is told he has no chance for recovery will become a chronic back cripple instead of a pro-ductive employee. Changing a patient's negative expectation is the most important thing the doctor can do.

When the doctor is convinced that sending a patient back to work with a sore neck or back is a dangerous thing to do, the doctor won't make the rec-ommendation. It just won't happen. Some physicians worry that they might be sued if the patient goes back to work and gets into trouble. To give the patient a positive message about going back to work, the clinician must be certain it is the right thing to do. If the doctor doesn't believe in the impor-tance of work for the good of the patient, the patient won't believe it either.

I am convinced that getting someone out of the house or out of the clinic and back into a normal daily routine, including work, is an essential part of recovery. But it is a very tough sell. Patients are quick to believe that they are being pushed to work for someone else's financial gain, perhaps to save the insurance company money or to serve the employer's need. Patients are often reluctant to accept that anyone considers their interests or that anyone could actually believe going to work is a good thing for them, not for someone else. I believe it is. I do my best to convince my patients to try. I have seen too many people who have failed and whose personalities have been swallowed up by victimhood. There is a need to act quickly. Your chance of returning to your regular occupation on a full-time basis drops by nearly 50 per cent after only six months of neck or back disability. Some studies suggest that after two years off work, you have no chance at all of getting back to your old job. This is not just a function of you and your pain. Times change, companies re-organize, and chances are lost. The statistic is frightening, but it makes sense.

After being injured at work, some people enter the world of compensation, expecting a financial reward: "I've paid into the system for years. It's time I got my money back."

It doesn't work that way. Compensation and disability payments are not like contributions to a retirement savings plan. The money may be available if you are injured, but it comes with strict regulations and definite time limits. That fact becomes ever clearer as the months pass. There is increasing pressure to resolve the problem and get back to work. Hostility grows. Litigation commences, and the opportunity for a productive working life is gone. There is no pot of gold at the end of the rainbow, no financial reward to compensate for a lifetime of lost earnings and lost opportunities.

I have seen too many tragic endings. I know that returning to work with pain is the right thing to do. It brings the short-term benefits of a sense of well-being and greater pain control. It delivers a greater long-term gift: the return to a normal life.

# CHAPTER FOURTEEN

## *Spine Care Made Easy*

Phineas T. Barnum, often regarded as America's greatest showman, lived by his own maxim, "There's a sucker born every minute." I am always disappointed when his words ring true in the world of spine care. Our technology is constantly opening doors to avenues that will lead us forward in our conquest of back and neck pain. But it also opens doors onto blind alleys where charlatans wait to prey upon the unsuspecting, eating their time and money. If you have chosen to begin our consultation here, looking for the shortcut to spine care, I've caught you. Spine care is not easy, but it is simple. And it is a partnership. Caring for your back or neck is your responsibility, and anyone who says otherwise is probably trying to sell you something.

I can't lay all the blame on those who offer magic solutions. Any successful confidence scheme must have a mark: someone who is willing to suspend rational thought in the hope that, this time, it will really work. Because back and neck pain are nearly universal, and because they apparently respond to so many different things, fraudulent claims are easy to make and difficult to disprove. All the more so because patients want to believe.

I recall a patient who came to see me two or three times with uncomplicated mechanical low back pain. His symptoms responded to a simple program for a Pattern 1 fast responder. I provided the necessary education, offered my support, and prescribed the appropriate series of treatment sessions. But that is not what he wanted. He had heard from a friend that injecting an anaesthetic into the painful lump he felt in his back at the top of his buttock would solve his problem. It had worked for her, so why wouldn't it work for him?

I explained that the lump (doctors call them fibrocytic nodules) was one of the body's non-specific responses to his underlying structural pain. Anaesthetizing the lump would be like blowing the smoke away from a fire. It would produce some temporary comfort, but it couldn't last. My patient's mind was made up, though. He had no interest in my other options, and so he demanded that I give him what he wanted.

Trigger-point injection, as the technique is called, is a safe, well-established procedure. I use it occasionally to give patients with those tender lumps the temporary relief they need to embark on a more lasting solution. I am reluctant to resort to trigger-point injections when I believe the needle is all the patient wants.

Recognizing that I was not going to change his mind, and to escape from his repeated demands, I agreed to give him the injection. I promised him nothing more than a short, pain-free interlude, but I was wrong. The injection worked, and it worked dramatically. His pain was gone and, with no further effort, his life returned to normal. I have no idea how the injection could have worked so well. Did it break a pain cycle that relieved other areas of muscle tension? Had it affected the gates to his pain-sensing system in the spinal cord? Whatever the reason, there was no doubt of its success. We parted company on the best of terms.

About a year later, I received a telephone call from a physician in Florida. He had recently seen a patient from Canada who came to his office complaining of low back pain and, in particular, a very painful lump at the top of his buttock. It was my former patient, and he had told the doctor of my injection and its miraculous result. The doctor hadn't heard of any drug available in the United States that could produce such a dramatic effect. He had called to inquire what I had used and whether there was any way he could obtain a sample. I could feel his disappointment, or perhaps it was his embarrassment, when I told him that my injection had been nothing but a long-acting local anaesthetic available all over the world.

For every patient who gets a good result from a trigger-point injection, there are dozens more who gain relief only for the time it takes for the local anaesthetic to dissipate, or who gain no benefit at all. One of the keys to a durable spine program is reliability. Mechanical spine pain will respond predictably to a physical treatment selected on the basis of the correct pattern. This obvious and open approach is more certain, efficient, and cost-effective than most of the highly publicized medicinal options or the mysterious secret remedies.

### You have said that back/neck pain often gets better by itself. Would I be just as well-off doing nothing?

If you have the knowledge and confidence to let nature take its course, that may be a reasonable approach. But many patients can't or won't put in the time. They want something done and they want it done in a hurry. Simply telling a patient to wait and see seldom works. While it can be good advice, it conveys the wrong impression that the doctor has no idea what to do and no idea what may happen. Patients are not fond of the thought that their health-care practitioner knows no more about the problem than they do. How much confidence would you have in the refrigerator technician who says, "I haven't got the faintest idea what's wrong here. What do you think we should try?"

When I am convinced that a patient's mechanical neck or back pain will get better with time and little else, I do not prescribe costly treatments or powerful drugs, but I do not just say, "Wait and see," either. There is always something the patient can do. With the pattern as a guide, treatment may speed recovery.

"I just wasted a visit with the therapist. She didn't do anything."

"She didn't take your history or examine you?"

"Well, she did that."

"And didn't she tell you what was wrong?"

"She said I had some kind of pattern thing and gave me some simple stretches and told me to sit with a pillow in the small of my back. But she didn't do anything."

I hear this kind of conversation all the time. Patients come looking for the magic touch, the "machine that goes ping," or the wonder drug. All they get is an answer, some education, and specific techniques to stop the pain, and that is not enough to satisfy them. Spine care can be so simple that sometimes it needs to be dressed up a little to be made believable. There is nothing wrong with that, as long as the underlying mechanical approach is sound, and the fancy clothes don't cost very much.

### Is identifying the patient's pattern of pain that important?
I believe it is. Spine care has progressed well past the point where everybody gets the same therapy. The more precise our treatment strategy becomes, the greater the need for an accurate diagnosis. Conservative management is not all that different from surgery. A successful operation requires that I know exactly where to go and what to cut. Successful non-operative care requires application of the right mechanical approach to the correct condition. Identifying the pattern of neck or back pain is the necessary first step. A spine-care program doesn't work well if you are using the wrong treatment for a particular type of spine pain, or if you are treating pain that isn't coming from the spine at all.

### Are there other pain locations that can be confused with the spine?
Yes, there are. The sacroiliac joint discussed in Chapter 9 is one location. Two other frequently confused sites are the shoulder and the hip.

Separating neck-dominant pain from pain arising in the shoulder requires close observation. To make it more difficult, about two out of every ten people with neck pain also have shoulder trouble. The two pains can co-exist. The pain from a sore neck can occasionally be felt in exactly the same location as the pain from a sore shoulder. Most of the time, if you are careful, you can tell the two of them apart. Here is a simple test you can try. If the pain is on the left side of your neck, take your right hand and cover the most painful area. For the other side, use your other hand. Where did you place your palm? If it is over or just below the point of your shoulder, the pain is probably coming from the shoulder joint itself. If your palm is resting between your neck and your shoulder in the area of your collarbone, your shoulder pain is probably coming from your neck. Pain radiating along the muscle ridge at the top of the shoulder is one of the commonest sites of referred neck-dominant pain.

Another way to tell where the pain originates is to see what happens when you move things. Most neck pain is Pattern 1. The typical pain is intensified as you flex your head forward and try to put your chin on your chest. Most shoulder pain comes from an irritation at the top of the joint under the bony shelf that forms your shoulder tip. Lift your arm straight out to the side and then try to raise it over your head. That usually causes the most pain. Another movement that hurts a sore shoulder is rotation. Start with your arm at your side, your elbow bent and your palm up as if you were holding a tray. Now rapidly move your hand back and forth from the front of your body out to the side. If the trouble is in your shoulder and not your neck both these shoulder movements should produce your typical pain. If you are still confused, you may be one of those people who have both.

Hip pain is frequently confused with low back pain. Pattern 1 and Pattern 2 back pain can both be felt on the outer aspect of the hip and into the groin. Hip pain can also spread to the groin, but it usually radiates further down the inner side of the thigh, and is occasionally more intense around the knee. Most orthopaedic surgeons can tell stories about a patient (always someone else's) who had an arthroscopy for a painful knee only to have the surgeon discover that the pain was coming from the hip. Although hip pain can spread to the outer aspect of the hip and into the buttock, pain in these two locations is much more likely to be coming from the back.

If you lie on your back and draw the knee on the painful side toward your stomach, you can test whether or not your pain is coming from the hip joint. With the knee and hip both bent at about ninety degrees, turn your lower leg outward, moving your foot away from the mid-line of your body. With your hip flexed this rotation puts the greatest stretch on the hip capsule and generally reproduces the typical hip pain.

A large soft-tissue pouch under the skin and covering the side of the hipbone, the trochanteric bursa, further complicates locating the pain source. The trochanter is a large bony prominence at the top of the thigh bone. A bursa is a fluid-filled sac that serves as a lubricating mechanism in parts of the body where adjoining tissues move in very different directions. When a bursa becomes inflamed, you have bursitis ("itis" = inflammation). Bursitis is painful. An inflamed trochanteric bursa is in exactly the same site as referred pain from the back. Confusing referred back pain and bursitis may be one reason why repeated cortisone injections into the bursa to reduce inflammation sometimes fail to stop the pain.

Someone with a bad back can also have pain in the hip. I saw a patient like that: the father of one of the physiotherapists working at CBI. His back pain was so bad that he had been forced to limit all his activities and he was barely able to continue working in his own business. When I first saw him, he was walking toward my office, slowly and obviously in pain. I was impressed by how stiff his gait seemed and how little he appeared to swing his legs. I started my physical examination on his hips, not on his back. Both hips had only a few degrees of movement and the flexion/rotation test I just described for demonstrating hip pain produced his typical symptoms. His problem was advanced osteoarthritis, which I successfully managed by replacing both hips with artificial joints. His life has returned to normal and, as it turns out, he did not have a bad back after all.

For patients who do have both hip and back pain, it is usually a good idea to correct the hip problem first. A modern hip replacement is a remarkably successful operation. Spine surgery is not always so predictable.

### I guess surgery is less successful the longer you have had the problem?

The duration of your pain is not as important as the duration of your disability: the length of time your back or neck problem has kept you from work and your normal activities. Some people have back or neck pain intermittently their whole lives and never need any treatment at all. Then the pain changes and the clinical picture indicates there is now a problem that requires surgical intervention. The duration of the previous, non-disabling pain will have no adverse effect on the outcome of the operation. When the pain begins to limit function, stop work, and prevent everyday movement, the situation begins to change. The longer the disability persists, the greater the danger that the individual will develop pain-focused behaviour. It can happen in months. Abnormal pain behaviour can destroy any chance of a successful surgery.

The problems I treat, either surgically or with education and exercise, are the ones you have right now. There is no evidence that something you did thirty years ago has any relationship to your present pain. Many patients are told that contact sports in high school are the cause of their neck pain at age fifty. There is absolutely no evidence this is true. You can't blame the back pain you are suffering as an adult on falling off the front porch and landing on your bottom when you were twelve. Many people carry this misplaced recrimination, and it fosters the belief that the back and neck are fragile and vulnerable structures.

**But you said mechanical spine pain is the result of the things we do to our backs and necks all through our lives?**
That's true. The pain comes from the accumulated effect of all that physical abuse plus the normal changes that accompany advancing maturity. Your spine is no more at risk than any of your other joints and, in many ways, it is better protected. The amount of pain you feel bears little relationship to the magnitude of the physical problem. Still, that comforting thought doesn't diminish the severity of an attack. For years, I told patients that if they had to face a dangerous situation such as escaping from a burning building, their back spasm would not prevent them from running. From everything I had learned and from my own experience, I was sure I was correct.

My attitude changed a little following a ski trip a few winters ago. My back had been bad for several months and, in spite of my back care and regular exercise, it kept right on hurting. I discovered how little sympathy you get when you are a back doctor with a sore back. My ski trip had been planned for some time and I have never been one to let my back tell me what to do, so I went. I was holding up reasonably well until the end of the first day. I was coming down a narrow track with a fairly steep pitch when

I came to a sharp bend. The trees were just ahead so I started my turn. Or at least, I tried to start. My legs were willing, but my back utterly refused. I tried to explain that not turning could have disastrous consequences but my back was adamant that a sudden twist would just be too painful. I made the turn with a complete lack of style and grace, but here I am. I still tell patients that in a dangerous situation, their back won't stop them from doing what has to be done. But now I add that they will have to be quite firm in their directions and be prepared for a dispute. That ski episode also reinforces the importance of knowing that, however much it may hurt, what you do cannot damage your back. Of course, without the confidence that knowledge provides, you probably would not have gone skiing in the first place. I think that would be the biggest mistake of all.

### You mentioned you were exercising with your sore back. Didn't that make the pain worse?

It may hurt to start, but for many people, exercise reduces the pain. The more you move, the better it feels. At the beginning of an attack, you are better to keep moving than to lie still and wait to see what happens. I am sure that I have prevented a number of my own attacks from worsening with early stretching and the pain-control movements. There may even have been times I stopped an attack before it started.

Acting early has another benefit. It offsets one of the body's responses to injury: oedema. When tissue is damaged, it allows fluid to leak out through the walls of the blood vessels into the spaces between the muscles. This is not the same as a bruise where blood flows out. This is a clear, sticky fluid that carries many necessary repair materials. If it stays very long, it can glue the tissues together. Spill a can of pop on the pages of a book (but not this one!). If you clean it off right away, the book's owner may never notice. If you let the pop dry, the pages will stay stuck together. Oedema does the same thing to the tissues in your body. Getting rid of oedema in the tissues means movement, and the sooner you start to move, the better. Wearing a cervical collar after the soft-tissue injury that occurs with whiplash allows the oedema to remain and unwanted stiffness to develop.

**Are the exercises you are talking about just stretches, or are there more?**

I divide exercise into two groups. The first are the simple stretches, not really exercises at all, that help in rapid pain control. The remaining ones are real exercises to strengthen muscles and improve endurance. I will discuss those in chapters 15 and 16. I recommend you begin an exercise program before you reach middle age. It's not that exercise in the elderly doesn't work; it does. There is a large body of evidence showing that active exercise programs can be effective. They can improve strength and increase muscle bulk into your seventies and eighties. But starting to exercise as an established senior citizen is a daunting challenge. Picture your great-aunt Dorothy: round and soft and sweet, and with no exercise experience. Where do you start? How do you explain that being out-of-breath right now and sore tomorrow morning is good for her? With no point of reference, she is not likely to join the fitness club.

You must decide for yourself whether you continue your exercises on a regular basis or not. Most people who try to exercise regularly succeed for a few months, or even a few years, before something breaks the routine. That's okay. Although it may be difficult to summon up the discipline to start again after a long absence, the benefits can be recovered and, like riding a bicycle, you never completely forget. Your neck and back pain will probably be less troublesome as you grow older and your spine gets stiffer. Still, that is a poor excuse for doing nothing right now. Nature may be on your side but it moves very slowly.

I can remember when I was a boy our family outings were often cancelled at the last moment because of my father's back problems. He would simply take to his bed. Years later, when I got into the business of telling people about back pain, I often said that most backs gets better with age. I said so in my first book. When *The Back Doctor* was published, my eighty-year-old father called me up and said, "I don't think it's right for you to go around saying things like that without consulting your dad."

"Okay," I said, "what happened to your back pain?'

"Well," he said, "it got better."

Our church just got a new minister. When I met him, I had the strange sense I'd seen him before. We looked at each other and both realized he had been a patient of mine twenty-five years earlier. He had seen me for his bad back. He recalled that I had told him he had the back of a ninety-year-old. I don't remember saying that, but knowing that backs get better with age, perhaps I meant it as encouragement. In any event, he had continued an active lifestyle, including basketball and weight training. Twenty-five years later, he told me his back was fine but his knees had worn out.

A commitment to exercise doesn't suit everyone. My dad was an active businessman and as a young man had been a sailor and a boxer. In his later years he was not interested in exercise and his back got better on its own. Our new minister took a different path and reached the same objective. Exercise is certainly helpful and I prescribe it regularly. But like all the other options in this business, the choice is up to you.

Exercise also has an important place in the management of the pain-focused patient. A recent study by British investigators showed a significant improvement in the symptoms of fibromyalgia in a group of patients taking regular aerobic exercise classes compared with those in relaxation sessions. The exercise group rated themselves as "much better" or "very much better" nearly twice as often, and at the end of one year had a statistically lower incidence of the typical characteristics of the condition.

## Can I exercise on my own, or do I need equipment?

The results you get from your exercise program will be in direct proportion to the amount of effort you put in. The harder you work, the stronger you become. For all the hype about one exercise machine versus another, you are still the ultimate limiting factor. No matter how hard you try, you may never look like the beautiful, buffed people in the ads, but exercise equipment does have its place, as long as your expectations are realistic and you don't plan to have the machine exercise for you. The standard sit-up is an excellent exercise for strengthening your upper abdomen. Many people with Pattern 1 back pain find the sit-up uncomfortable because it diminishes their lumbar lordosis and loads the disc. Many others find it painful to rock back and forth on their tailbone. Any piece of equipment that maintains the curve in your low back and cushions your tailbone is helpful. They may not make you look like a body-builder, but they can let you exercise in comfort.

One of the most important advances in exercise training for low back pain is the increased emphasis on strengthening the muscles that run along your spine, the paraspinal muscles. The traditional exercise was to lie on your stomach and arch your back by raising your head and shoulders off the ground. This could be alternated with lifting both legs backward through the hips. The very fit elevated shoulders and legs at the same time. One problem with that exercise is that it recruits a large number of muscle groups, all the way from the muscles in the back of your neck and shoulders to the muscles in the back of your thighs. Your spinal muscles, the ones that need the work, get too much help. Because they require you to arch your back acutely, many patients with slow-responding Pattern 1 or Pattern 2 can't do these exercises at all.

For paraspinal strengthening, a simple piece of exercise equipment is very helpful. Most fitness clubs have a unit often called a "Roman chair." I have no idea where the name comes from. I doubt that any Roman ever sat on a chair that looked like one of these things. You lie on your stomach on an inclined frame that supports you up to your waist. Your ankles and lower legs are held in place, allowing you to bend forward so that your upper body is hanging down. The difficulty of the exercise is changed by adjusting the angle of the lower body support. The more it approaches the vertical, the easier the exercise becomes. Flexing forward at the waist and then coming up again works the muscles along your spine. Because of the equipment's design, the other muscle groups are hardly involved. You can isolate the paraspinal muscles in your low back and force them to do the work.

There are many different designs of exercise equipment. They all do about the same thing. Some have elaborate computer-based measuring systems. Others are about as sophisticated as your ironing board. With a little ingenuity, you could build one yourself. The point of the equipment is to make the exercise more valuable: that should always be its role.

Equipment can magnify the effect of your exercise. If you do everything right, a machine can increase your benefits. But if you do everything wrong, the machine may only magnify your pain. One example is the leg-press machine. It is designed to strengthen the muscles in your thighs. Although there are several variations, most units have you sit on a small seat with your knees bent and your feet resting on a bar or a pair of pedals. Pushing against a predetermined amount of resistance, you slowly straighten your legs then gradually bend them back to the starting point. Sometimes there is seat belt to help you maintain your position. Sometimes there is a back support to help you maintain correct spinal posture. But nowhere is there anything to prevent you from arching your back to help your legs when the weight gets too high. If you are a Pattern 1 slow responder or a Pattern 2, that can hurt. It all comes down to technique.

Sometimes you may not even be aware of the problem. At one time, I used a machine to exercise my biceps. I would sit on a stool with my arms forward and the back of my upper arms resting on a sloping surface. With my elbows bent, I could reach a bar. I drew it toward me by flexing my elbows. Increasing the weight increased the difficulty. Often during my circuit in the gym, I would develop a nasty headache. I tried to improve my breathing, the order of the exercises, and the length of the program. Nothing helped. Then, one day, one of the staff noticed that as I was working on my biceps, I was thrusting my head forward. It was a simple question of posture correction. I regularly teach the importance of keeping your head back as you lift. I totally overlooked keeping my own head back on that machine.

### What about exercises without equipment? Aquatic exercise, for example?

I consider a swimming pool to be a rather expensive piece of exercise equipment, but that's not the point. Exercising in the water can be very worthwhile. You put your muscles through their paces while the effect of gravity is neutralized by your buoyancy in the water. You can gain all the benefits of stretching, strengthening, and an aerobic routine while keeping the load off your spine. A well-designed pool program is an excellent form of therapy.

I have two minor reservations when my patients tell me that they have started swimming to help their backs. Swimming will help them only if they follow a schedule of exercises. Just getting into the water and bobbing around is not enough. Like using a piece of dry-land exercise equipment, you still have to do the work. It may be difficult to stick to the routine. Some patients who start pool therapy in a rehabilitation department do well until they are discharged, then drop out because they do not have easy access to another suitable location. Some fitness clubs, community centres, and parks have pools. So do many private residences. But having water available is only the first step. You need a routine, a schedule, and, often, some supervision. Going in alone may not give you as much of a workout as playing with the children. The pool only adds an element of protection. It is the exercise that helps, not the healing waters.

### What about aerobic exercise?
Aerobics these days are "low impact." They are certainly excellent for your heart and lungs. To gain the most benefit, they should be combined with a stretching routine. I think aerobics are at their best when added to a strength-training program. Increasing muscle mass is actually another way of improving your aerobic capacity. Jogging and speed-walking are excellent aerobic exercises. So is working out on an exercise bicycle, a stair climber, or a ski machine. The way you get your aerobic input will depend on what's available and on whether you prefer the rain or the television in your face.

### How about yoga or Tai Chi?
They are certainly not fads. Both have been around for centuries. Tai Chi is considered a form of the Oriental martial arts, although the current emphasis is on a series of slow and gentle movements. The routines last from ten minutes to half an hour and stress balance, co-ordination, and relaxation. The discipline trains motion coming from the "core" of the body (the abdomen and back), not from the external parts such as the arms and shoulders. The movements are mostly circular and of an even tempo concentrating on balance and a smooth weight shift from one side of the body to the other. Tai Chi has gained adherents around the world as a healthy combination of exercise and mental concentration.

Like Tai Chi, yoga exercises are not directed primarily at strength, although they are more strenuous. The focus is flexibility. The physical aspects of yoga (the name comes from Sanskrit, the language of India's ancient religious texts) are said to have been developed as a vehicle for meditation, creating the necessary stamina for the mind to remain calm. The various positions may prepare your body for stillness but whether they can actually increase the range of movement in your back is questionable. Some of us simply have to live with our stiff spines. Years ago someone decided that yoga would be a good exercise for everyone working at the CBI corporate office. I remember the first session. The instructor asked me to sit on the floor with my legs spread wide apart and straight out in front of me. Then I was to gently place my forehead on my knee. I could look down at my knee from a great height, but that wasn't good enough. In spite of her attempts to physically assist me, that was the only view I ever got. I noticed other staff having a similar problem. Shortly after that, someone decided that yoga was not the way for us to go.

There is also some evidence from research with ballet dancers that increased flexibility of the spine offers no protection from back injury. Studies have suggested that there is an equal number of problems in the group whose spines are more flexible than average and the group with less flexibility than normal. And, of course, no one can agree on exactly what normal is.

Yoga and Tai Chi both offer relaxation and breathing exercises. These are excellent methods of achieving temporary pain control. If stretching feels good, then stretch. If you, like me, never get your forehead near your knee, don't worry.

As with any activity, you might be wise to adapt your Tai Chi or yoga exercises to your particular pattern of pain. If flexion is the thing that hurts, then limit or modify any position or stretch that requires too much forward-bending. But don't confuse the pull of tight muscles with the onset of your typical pain. Don't be afraid to try.

### Are there other exercise options?

Similar but considerably more recent approaches to the mind-body relationship can be found in eponymous exercise routines such as the Alexander Technique, or the Pilates or Feldenkrais Methods.

The Alexander Technique, originated by Frederick Alexander, concentrates on balance, posture, breathing, and co-ordination. It strives to release unnecessary and unconscious muscle tension by changing the ways followers sit, stand, walk, or participate in other daily activities. Proponents consider it more than a series of exercises; it is a re-education of the mind and body. A variation of the technique called the Mitzvah Exercise was designed to "ripple the spine upward." It claims that, "as the head frees on top of the spine, the rest of the body realigns and rebalances while correcting itself all the way down to the toes."

The Pilates Method of physical and mental conditioning was developed by Joseph Pilates and first gained popularity as a form of dance training. The basic principles integrate improved body alignment, breathing, and efficiency of motion. A sequence of precise, carefully performed movements, each associated with a specific breathing pattern, releases tension by stretching and strengthening selected muscles. Some of the exercises require specially designed equipment. The method demands more personal supervision than most other exercise programs.

The Feldenkrais Method was created by Dr. Moshe Feldenkrais. The moves, taught in one-to-one sessions or small classes, train the participants to correct posture for improved movement and flexibility. The method focuses on small, precise movements that can be practised any time during the day. It professes to offer an "incredibly relaxing principle" that has mental as well as physical benefits.

All of these routines have similar characteristics emphasizing posture, muscle control, and relaxation. All assume a mind-body connection. Some are more strenuous and technically demanding, but their intent is the same: to overcome stress and restore a healthy balance to the body. These are admirable goals, but ones that do not necessarily require such esoteric approaches. Just identifying a pattern of pain and the movements that control it may be a place to start.

## You have made the patterns of pain very clear-cut. Can you always identify a pattern?

The clarity of the patterns is the result of the contributions of many clinicians working at CBI. It is the patterns' precise definition that has allowed them to serve as a basis for our neck and back treatment program and as templates for the management of other musculoskeletal complaints. And no, it isn't always possible to identify a pattern. Sometimes being unable to identify one means you are dealing with a non-mechanical neck or back problem. The inability to establish a pattern or the lack of an anticipated response to a specific treatment should alert you to a potential problem. Using pattern recognition rather than memorizing a lengthy list of possible causes of spinal pain is a safe and effective shortcut to diagnosis.

But sometimes even when the problem is only mechanical, the patterns can be difficult to identify. Here are two examples.

You see a seventy-year-old man who complains of pain in his legs when he walks. After five minutes both his legs begin to feel rubbery and weak. They start to ache and he is forced to sit down to relieve the symptoms. After a few minutes of sitting, his legs feel fine. But as he is sitting his back starts to hurt. By the time his legs are feeling better, his back pain is almost intolerable. The only way he can get relief is to stand up. Once he is standing, the back pain starts to subside. He tells you that as far as his back is concerned, he would rather walk than stand and he would much rather stand than sit down. When you question him about the site of his dominant pain (the first and most important question) he simply cannot decide. His legs are bad but so is his back. Both pains are intermittent. What pattern would you choose? One of the guides is that, when you cannot choose between back and leg pain, the leg symptoms should take precedence. The man's leg symptoms are clearly Pattern 4. His back pain is just as clearly Pattern 1. Some patients do exhibit more than one pattern, and sometimes both can be an ordeal.

For the second case you see a thirty-two-year-old woman with a two-year history of constant, left-leg-dominant pain. Her pain is worse when she sits or bends forward. She does have pain in her low back and buttock, but there is no question in her mind that her leg pain is her major problem.

When you examine her, there is no evidence of nerve-root irritation and all the neurological tests are normal. What pattern would you choose? Part of the story sounds like Pattern 1. But the pain is leg-dominant. Part of the story sounds like Pattern 3, but without evidence of direct nerve-root involvement, that option is not available. Patterns 2 and 4 are always intermittent, and this pain is constant.

Both of these cases are the stories of real patients. The first man responded to an abdominal-strengthening program and posture correction for his Pattern 4 leg pain. However, his back pain got worse as his leg pain got better. The flexed posture he needed to help his legs aggravated his discs. In the end, the program didn't satisfy his needs and so I operated. I decompressed his spinal canal and fused one level. The physical source of his problem was degenerative spondylolisthesis, where one bone slips in relation to another. Although it is more common in women, it does happen in men. His back-dominant pain resulted from the loss of mechanical stability. His leg pain with walking occurred because of the narrowing of the space for the nerves as the ring of the spinal canal above slid past the ring of the canal below. Both problems were corrected at surgery and his final result was excellent.

In listening to the young woman's history, I became convinced that her problem was an unusual presentation of Pattern 1. I thought her pain sounded mechanical and I suspected it arose in the discs. With further questioning, she told me that two years earlier, when the pain started, her leg pain was much more intense. For several weeks, the constant leg pain had been so bad that it was impossible for her to lift her left leg. I think that two years ago, she had acute sciatica (Pattern 3) caused by direct pressure from a disc on one of the nerves running into her left leg. That period of nerve compression and inflammation increased the nerve's ability to transmit pain, rendering it more sensitive and irritable. The bulging disc was no longer irritating the nerve, but the bulge itself continued to hurt: the outer shell is very responsive to distortion. Now, although the dominant pain should have been in her back, that sensitized nerve was carrying the pain message down the same well-worn track. Her back-dominant pain of Pattern 1 was being referred so strongly that her leg hurt more than her spine.

I asked her to lie on her stomach on the examining table and taught her how to do a sloppy push-up. After ten repetitions, her leg pain had begun to subside. I left her resting on her stomach and went to see another patient. When I returned, I asked her to do ten more push-ups. Before she left the clinic after her first visit, her constant left leg pain had disappeared completely. She was pain-free. Her response to my treatment, which was based on the presumption of Pattern 1, was excellent. I could explain her unusual presentation from her history. I could rule out active nerve-root involvement from her physical examination. And I could test my hypothesis about her pattern through her response to therapy. More importantly, I produced her first period of complete pain relief in two years.

### So recognizing the correct pattern isn't as easy as it sounds?

Recognizing the pattern can be tricky. It takes practice. To improve skills, we regularly prepare sample cases to test the clinicians at CBI. Here are a couple of recent examples. See how you do.

A sixty-year-old woman arrives in the clinic with a chief complaint of headache. She describes her pain as beginning in the back of her neck at the base of her skull and then spreading to an area behind both eyes. The pain always starts on the left side. Sometimes it is so severe that she feels nauseous.

Her headaches can last for a week at a time. They are usually worse in the morning and when she has to drive for more than an hour. When she has no headache, she still feels pain in her neck that runs down between her shoulder blades and sometimes up along her jaw. The pain increases when she looks down.

The physical examination shows normal power in both arms, but there are no reflexes on either side. The neurological examination of the legs is normal, although the reflexes are difficult to obtain.

The answer is Pattern 1 neck pain. Headache is one of the common referral sites and the symptoms are aggravated by forward head posture, lying on a poor pillow, and driving. The reflexes are absent on both sides and a symmetrical loss with no other neurological findings is not significant. Too easy? Try the next one.

This patient is a fifty-three-year-old woman whose doctor sent her to the clinic with a chief complaint of pain when walking. She says that her pain begins when she walks for half the length of the shopping mall and that it will not stop until she sits down and bends forward. It feels better to rest her elbows on her knees. Once the pain is gone, she can walk again but only for the same distance.

The physical examination finds that both her ankle reflexes are absent. The straight leg-raise test gives her pain when either leg is lifted to about sixty degrees.

The doctor who referred her for treatment had already obtained a CT scan of her lumbar spine. The X-rays show marked narrowing of the spinal canal caused by severe degenerative changes in the small spinal joints. What pattern have you selected? If you have chosen any pattern at all, you've made a mistake. Go back and look at the history again. The site of the dominant pain is never mentioned. Without that vital piece of information, you cannot pick a pattern.

On further questioning, she tells you that her pain is in her low back and buttocks. Occasionally it spreads to her groin but it never runs down her legs. The pain is Pattern 2, intermittent and aggravated by the natural arching of the back that occurs when we walk on flat surfaces. The narrowed spinal canal on X-ray has no bearing on the patient's symptoms. Although the nerves are compressed, they are functioning normally and require no treatment.

As this case shows, selecting the correct pattern of pain demands careful attention to all the details. It requires taking a careful history, whether you are listening to someone else or taking it on yourself. But once you have identified the pattern of pain and confirmed it with the physical examination, selecting the proper treatment should be almost automatic. The probability of success is extremely high. Maybe "Spine Care Made Easy" is the right title for this chapter after all.

# CHAPTER FIFTEEN

## *Gym Class*

I have a copy of a book on medical-mechanical therapy written by Dr. Gustif Zander, professor of medical gymnastics. The book was published in 1880. That was nearly thirty years after Dr. Max Hurz wrote his book, illustrated with an impressive array of exercise machines and equipment for treating back and neck pain and a variety of other musculoskeletal complaints. Exercise is not a new strategy. But its applications change as our understanding improves. We have already separated out those easily performed activities that hasten pain control. These are better described as movements or postures rather than exercises and they are directly related to the pattern of pain. They are intended only as a strategy for the prompt relief of symptoms, not as a means of permanent control or even lasting comfort.

Strengthening exercises are largely independent of the patient's pain-producing movements, posture, or specific patterns. They are intended to strengthen the muscles that support the spine, enabling the former sufferer to maintain a posture or perform an activity in the most desirable way. Strong muscles don't stop pain, but they can limit its intensity. Proper body mechanics reduces the load on the spine and a reduced load on that sore "thing" in the neck or back means less pain. Many of the exercises I recommend today are the same exercises I recommended when I first started in practice. Most can be found in the pages of Dr. Hurz's or Dr. Zander's books. Although I didn't know it at the time, many of the exercises I believed to be recent innovations were merely returning to fashion. Extension exercises for the low back have enjoyed a recent wave of popularity but, like the abdominal-strengthening exercises that held sway before them, they have all been seen before. What has changed the most are the applications and the techniques. Pairing specific exercises with specific mechanical patterns seems obvious now, but it was revolutionary thirty years ago. Training techniques have introduced the concept of isolated muscle exercise. The goal of providing strength in the neck and shoulder girdle and muscular support to the trunk remains the same but the means to achieve it have significantly improved.

That does not mean that an existing program you find effective should be discarded. If it worked for you in the past, there is no reason to abandon it now. Some of the exercise programs in *The Back Doctor* seem as dated as the pictures in those old European exercise books. Nevertheless, over the years, I have had patient after patient assure me that they work. The fundamentals and the foundations have not changed. We have enlarged our exercise routines, not replaced them.

Sometimes I think we go a bit too far. In their effort to define the perfect exercise, some enthusiasts decide that weakness or decreased flexibility of a single muscle is the culprit. They devise routines that purport to strengthen a single unit while all its neighbours remain at rest. Such artificial precision is not possible, and it is not entirely harmless. One muscle frequently chosen for special training is the multifidis muscle along the spine. It is one of a series of muscles lying deep in the back adjacent to the vertebrae. All the members of the group (multifidis, semispinalis, and rotatores) share common attachments to adjacent portions of the vertebrae. The only difference between the members is the number of segments that they span. Multifidis covers an intermediate distance, less than the longer semispinalis and more than the shorter rotatores. As they travel together along the spine, they blend to form a single large muscle. Except by anatomical dissection, isolating multifidis is impossible. Approaching the spine surgically, there is no way to tell which muscle fibres are separated. Ignoring the fact that these three muscles are really different portions of the same structure, exercise consultants devise programs to strengthen only multifidis. Presumably, these routines leave the contiguous bands of muscle that surround it completely at rest. It makes no sense and is physiologically impossible. You may ask, "But what difference does that make? Isn't any exercise beneficial?"

Maybe so, but I still object to this approach. This spurious science accords unjustified value to a particular exercise routine, stamping it superior to a general fitness program. It is a marketing technique that enables some experts to be more "expert" than others and to charge correspondingly higher fees. It seems to confirm the concept that the spine is a highly complex, possibly delicate structure that must be treated with special care. Your inability to work only multifidis might even discourage you from using a less sophisticated routine in the belief that you would be wasting your time.

Simple ideas approached in a complicated manner become complicated. While exercise techniques can be improved and their results can be enhanced, the principle of exercise is simple and it should stay that way.

### How long will it take for your exercises to cure my back?

Whenever I hear a question like that I despair. These are not my exercises, and they will never "cure" your back. Exercise programs have evolved over time. The fashions may change, but the underlying principles remain the same. No one is in a position to lay claim to the concept of exercise. Exercise will never cure mechanical neck or back pain because there is no illness to attack.

The question "How long?" can be asked in two ways. How long will it take for exercise to demonstrate a positive effect? How long must I continue to exercise in order to keep my back and neck pain-free?

Exercise improves function in two ways. The training effect occurs early. It relates to the way you perform an exercise or use a piece of equipment. Your early gains may only reflect your improved physical skill. My personal example is the exercise ski machine. It looked so easy on television. My initial goal was a ten-minute routine but I couldn't complete a quarter of that. It wasn't lack of stamina so much as the fact that I kept falling off the skis. My improvement in the first week had nothing to do with improving aerobic capacity. It had everything to do with developing my timing and balance.

The second benefit of exercise comes from actual gains in strength and endurance. These things take time. Different muscle groups develop at different rates. It may be the way they are used, or something in the muscle fibres themselves, but there is no doubt that your biceps will enlarge long before your belly will flatten. Unfortunately, developing strength in the muscles of your neck and around your trunk is a slow process. I tell patients that the first three months of exercise should be considered an act of faith. They will see no change. Only after that will the effects start to become noticeable and finally offer visible encouragement and positive feedback. When you are in pain and anxious for help, three months is a very long time. Many patients, particularly those who have never tried to exercise before, just can't make it. They quit too soon. They come back looking for an alternative, but there isn't one.

I have a patient who continues to suffer back-dominant pain years after a simple decompression for Pattern 3 leg pain. His leg symptoms are gone but his back hurts. He is overweight, out-of-shape, and obsessed with his pain. He wants another operation to fix the problem. I have told him that I would not even consider a spinal fusion, the only surgical option, until he had been working out regularly and vigorously for at least six months. After that, we will talk. "Okay," he said. "I can try, but I know I'll fail. So can I just have my operation now?" He will never get a fusion, at least, not from me.

Still, exercise is not the answer for everyone. It may be a valuable option, but not in every case. Many people come to the CBI clinics for prompt control of their acute spine pain. They are successfully managed with a combination of education, activity adjustment, and simple pain-control activities. They never see the gym and they don't need to. They return to their normal activities pain-free but in the same physical condition in which they arrived. They will deal with the next attack when and if it happens. Exercise is most useful for back- and neck-pain sufferers whose work or lifestyle demands certain activities that are repeatedly or inevitably painful. Their only defence may be stronger muscles and exercise may be the best answer.

An occupational physician working with a group of mining companies recently asked me about the advisability of starting a back-exercise protocol in the mines. The target group was the men who drove the two-hundred-ton ore-moving trucks in and out of the pit. They routinely worked twelve-hour shifts, subjected to constant vibration and the repeated jolts of the rough roads. Most of them were about sixty years old, smoked, and were over-weight. But they enjoyed the work, earned a good wage, and reported almost no back pain. At first look, they were perfect subjects for a back-fitness program. But were they? Back pain was not a problem. And it was almost certain that the miners wouldn't finish their long shifts then head to the gym for a workout. Increasing the workers' awareness of back pain was more likely to create a problem than solve one. Not everyone needs to be in top shape to do the job. Just like prescribing needless medication or manipula-tion, recommending purposeless back exercise can do more harm than good.

### If I decide to start exercising, how long do I have to keep it up?

There is no time limit. As long as you want the benefit to continue, you have to keep on with your exercise. It is the same situation faced by people who want to lose weight. They attend special classes and go on special diets until they have shed enough pounds to reach their target. From then on, they are on their own. For some, as the enthusiasm fades, so does their self-restraint. They revert to their old habits and ways of eating. Their weight climbs right back to where it was. As long as you exercise, you will maintain your increased strength and muscle endurance. When you stop, it doesn't take long for your muscles to return to their old ways. Physiologists tell us that within six weeks from the time you stop, the major benefits of a weight-training program are largely gone.

### But that is a permanent commitment. Are you saying I will have to exercise every day for the rest of my life?

You are right; it is a long-term commitment, and not one that everyone will sustain. To make it even tougher, the changes come gradually at the beginning. I have never had a patient who said to me: "I remember that wonderful morning after I had been exercising for six months when I awoke to find myself pain-free and a perfect physical specimen." But patients do tell me that they feel better and that their back pain comes less often and strikes with less force. Some patients who gain these benefits decide that now they are feeling better, exercise is too much bother. Of course, once the exercise stops, so do its benefits. The good news is you lose nothing when you stop except the gains you made. Sometimes establishing that cause-and-effect relationship between exercise and pain relief is a necessary lesson.

And you will not have to exercise every day. To use a simplistic explanation, strength training works by slightly damaging your muscles. Responding to that injury, they strengthen and enlarge. Recovery takes time, so you should not vigorously attack the same muscle group again for a couple of days. Performing the same exercise routine every other day is actually more effective than repeating it on a daily basis. There is also a psychological benefit from having that break. These exercises require real effort and time and facing them can be intimidating. A day off in between can do wonders for your attitude.

If you want to exercise every day, set up two or three different routines that exercise different muscles. You can have your daily gym time without interruption and still give your muscles a chance to recover.

### How do I start?

Start slowly. If you have exercised in the past but have been away from it for a while, you will need to return gradually. You can't expect to begin at your previous level, particularly if it has been several years. At fifty, none of us have the stamina and strength we had when we were twenty, as much as we might pretend we do. If you have never exercised before, even the simplest routines may seem strange and uncomfortable. There is no hurry. Your back and neck pain are quite willing to wait. Remember that old saying, "A thousand-mile journey begins with a single step."

Once you are underway, you should progress gradually as well. Stay at the same level of activity for a couple of weeks before you move up. Pay attention to your technique. Five proper repetitions offer more benefit than twice that number done poorly. Don't rush, and avoid ballistic movements where you use speed, momentum, and the weight of your body to achieve the result. Trying to touch your toes slowly is very different from rocking rapidly back and forth trying to hurl your head at your feet.

### How much exercise will I need?

Everyone's requirements are different. Some lucky people need very little. It depends partly on where you start.

If you are already in good physical shape, gaining additional strength and endurance may require some effort. But once you reach your target, which is control of your neck and back symptoms, you need go no further. Unless you are planning to enter a body-building contest, how you look is less important than how you feel. Defining your muscles and taking an inch or two off your waist may be desirable side effects, but they are not your principal goal. Once your exercise program balances with the needs of your neck and back that is enough.

Exercise can seem addictive. Once you get started and have the habit, you just don't feel right without it. Because repetition improves your performance, your routine grows easier, so there is always a temptation to intensify the program. If a little is good, more is better. But pushing beyond the level you need for pain control has significant drawbacks. You started to exercise because of neck or back pain. If you push your spine too hard, the benefits of the exercise may be completely nullified by the return of the pain. And more exercise takes more time. Most of us have schedules that can accommodate only so much. Setting aside thirty minutes or an hour is possible. Two hours just can't be done, at least not on a regular basis. People continue to expand their programs until the time and energy required exceed what they can afford. At this point people don't cut down, they cut out. Somehow it is more natural to say, "This is too much. I quit," than to say, "This is too much. I think I will go back to my easier, shorter routine." If your exercise program fits your lifestyle and is making you feel better, leave it alone.

## Are there bad exercises, as well as good ones?

Most "bad" exercises are just inefficient. They take valuable time away from the routines that do more good. Inexperienced clinicians often make the mistake of prescribing more exercises for the patient who is having trouble doing one when what is really required is a review of technique. They seem to believe the patient's lack of progress will be solved by new exercises that will be done as poorly as the one that has already failed.

The clinician isn't solely to blame. Many patients, frustrated by their lack of improvement, demand something more be done. They will not be satisfied with a mere revision of what they already think they know. Six new exercises will keep the client happy and gives the illusion of progress. Even when additional exercises may be helpful and they are all performed correctly, too many exercises get in the way. There are several exercises to strengthen your lower abdominal muscles. Some, like a single straight leg lift, produce minimal effect. Lifting both legs together is both more difficult and more efficient. Asking a patient to do single lifts on each side then to lift both legs together takes up more time but adds virtually nothing to the result. Pick the exercise that pays the biggest return on your investment and stay with it. I am not impressed when patients proudly announce that their routines contain fifteen or twenty exercises. Done properly, that program would take most of the day. I know they don't spend that amount of time. Those patients and their therapists just don't get it.

Experience has taught me to be a little sceptical whenever a patient assures me that he or she is doing the exercises correctly but that they are not helping. Usually I ask for a little demonstration. Doing something regularly and doing it correctly are not the same thing.

There are a few exercises I suggest you avoid. One consists of rolling your head around and around in a circle from shoulder to shoulder. People imagine this is relaxing their neck muscles but all they are really doing is making themselves dizzy while trying to simulate the mechanism of a whiplash. I am surprised when anyone still uses that antiquated routine.

Deep-knee bends provide little added benefit and cause considerable discomfort. A deep-knee bend puts significant stress on the joint. If you are at a stage of advancing maturity where your back is starting to complain, it is very likely your knees won't be too happy, either. Knees are very sensitive to your body weight and to the strength in your thighs. Strong thigh muscles assist both your back and your legs. But a deep-knee bend does not strengthen the muscles any faster than a bend limited to ninety degrees. Placing your back against the wall, sliding down until your hips and knees are both at right angles, and then sitting there on that imaginary chair puts a lot less stress on the joints. It won't take long for your thigh muscles to tell you what they think.

The standard sit-up is very misunderstood exercise. It is an excellent way to strengthen the upper abdomen. Unfortunately, many people are told it is dangerous because of the load it applies to the discs. There is no doubt that biomechanically, the sit-up increases disc pressure, but there is no clinical evidence that it does any harm. I remember one Pattern 4 patient who had done extremely well with an abdominal strengthening routine that included sit-ups. His leg symptoms had virtually disappeared. One evening, he attended a lecture from a fitness expert, who informed the audience that the sit-up was one of the most dangerous exercises ever devised. Of course, my patient stopped his routine and, within two months, his leg pain had returned. When he told me that story, I asked him what problems he had been having with his back while he was exercising. He said there had been none. I recommended he resume his sit-ups. Two months later, his leg pain was gone again. Done properly for the right reasons, the sit-up is a very useful exercise.

The irony is that many people who are afraid to do sit-ups are told to do crunches instead. I have seen very few people who can do a proper slow crunch. Some of them simply throw their head and neck forward at the same time as they try to hurl their knees up onto their stomachs. That rapid ballistic movement gives people headaches. The crunch is every bit as hard on the discs as the old-fashioned sit-up. Most patients just lift their head and feet a few inches off the floor, using only the muscles in their shoulders and thighs. They don't get headaches and they don't exercise their abdomen. The crunch is as biomechanically challenging as the sit-up, but, unless it is performed correctly, it offers less benefit.

People are told that the sit-up is dangerous only when they come all the way to a sitting position. In fact, that is the least stressful position but it is also less efficient. When you're sitting all the way up, it is essentially a rest break. If you are serious about your sit-ups, hover with your shoulder blades off the floor and never sit up completely.

One of the common mistakes people make when they do sit-ups is to anchor their feet by hooking them under the edge of the couch or the bar on the exercise bench. With your feet held in place, the sit-up becomes an exercise for your thigh muscles. While your knees may benefit, your abdominal muscles will not be impressed. I remember a patient who bragged he was doing a hundred sit-ups a day. I asked him to demonstrate. He said, "Sure, just sit on my feet." When I refused, he barely managed five. I will always recall the medical student who told me it was physiologically impossible to perform a sit-up without having your feet held down. He couldn't do it, and he assumed no one else could either.

The whole idea is to select an exercise that strengthens a particular group of muscles without wasting your time or creating unnecessary physical strain. There is no perfect routine, but whatever you choose, it should make you feel better.

## Do you select specific exercises because of your pattern of pain?

Not to the same degree as the pain-control activities I discussed in Chapter 5. Most chronic neck and back pain benefits from uniform muscle strength. A few Pattern 1 patients will never be comfortable performing a sit-up, so they find other ways to strengthen the abdomen. A few patients with Pattern 2 will never enjoy an exercise that requires them to arch their spine. For them, strengthening the muscles along the back requires a different strategy.

Sometimes I select an exercise because it has particular merit for a specific pattern. Strengthening the paraspinal muscles in the low back for patients with chronic Pattern 1 low back pain is a good example. I am convinced that an isolated lumbar extension exercise is one of the most useful exercises we offer. There is some interesting research to support my view. A few studies suggest that as little as ten minutes a week of focused lumbar paraspinal muscle strengthening is an effective way to control back pain arising in the lumbar discs. Ten minutes a week isn't a very long time. Thirty lumbar extensions on a Roman chair take about three minutes. If you include that exercise in your program three times a week, you still have one minute to spare. It doesn't take very much of the correct exercise to make a difference.

I have divided the exercises into two groups: those for the neck and shoulder girdle and those for the low back and legs. I make only a few references to the patterns. By now you should be able to determine which of these exercises is most suitable for you. A balanced program seems profitable for most patients. I suggest that you review all the options before making your choices. This section contains the exercises that I have found most effective. There are certainly many others. You will probably want to mix and match to create your own program.

These are real exercises. If you are planning to work out at home, find a convenient space with adequate ventilation. Wear comfortable clothes that do not constrict your circulation and, for the sake of your friends and family, take a shower when you are through. The exercises are best done steadily to raise your heart rate and provide maximum cardiovascular benefit. Schedule time when you will not be disturbed. Make finishing the program without interruption a priority.

If you have not exercised before, or even if you have, you might be advised to check the program with your doctor. I am focusing here on exercises for your neck and back, but they will require you to place stress on the rest of your body as well. A history of heart problems or other medical difficulties may require that you modify your routine.

The pelvic tilt is not an exercise. It is frequently a starting position and it is a goal for patients with Pattern 4. In recent years, the pelvic tilt has fallen out of fashion with the renewed enthusiasm for extension exercise. It remains, however, a basic manoeuvre, and one that should be mastered as you proceed. Assuming a pelvic tilt while lying on your back is largely a question of technique. Holding a pelvic tilt when you stand up is definitely a matter of strength.

Start by lying on your back with your knees bent and your feet flat on the floor. Without holding your breath, tighten your abdominal muscles, roll your hips forward, and contract your buttocks. The idea is to flatten the small of your back. You can raise your buttocks slightly, although it is better if they do not leave the ground. Don't push with your feet. Lying with a pelvic tilt should not require a great deal of muscular effort. The position should feel comfortable for most people except perhaps for an acute Pattern 1 or Pattern 3. Use the pelvic tilt to start all the flexion strengthening exercises.

Your exercise session can last anywhere from twenty minutes to an hour. The same routine should be repeated on alternate days. It's up to you how long you work out and how hard you push yourself. As your favourite teacher told you years ago, "You will only get out of the lesson what you put into it."

## NECK AND SHOULDER GIRDLE EXERCISES

### Neck Exercise #1: The Shrug

Stand or sit in a relaxed fashion with your arms hanging at your sides. Raise your shoulders as high as you can toward your ears. This action uses the muscles of your shoulder girdle that suspend your collar bones and your shoulder blades. They are the muscles that stabilize the base of your neck.

Keep your head well-balanced and avoid thrusting your chin forward.

Shrug your shoulders up and hold them for a slow count of five. Let them drop and then repeat. Ten repetitions is a reasonable place to start.

This exercise is more valuable if the shrugs are performed while you hold weights in your hands. Select a comfortable amount of weight. Limit the movement to the muscles across the tops of your shoulders. Avoid moving your head. Perfect your technique before you increase the weight.

### Neck Exercise #2: Resisted Retraction

This is an isometric exercise. The word isometric describes a method of exercise in which one set of muscles is tensed and held against the action of an opposing set of muscles. Charles Atlas called it "dynamic tension."

The muscles in your neck tense against the muscles in your arms. Done properly, there is no movement and your head remains completely still. If you increase the pressure too much, you will start to tremble. That may reawaken your pain and it makes the exercise less effective.

Start by putting your hands behind your head and lace your fingers together. Push back with your head as you pull forward with your arms. Hold the pressure for a slow count of five and then relax. Ten repetitions is a reasonable goal. As your strength improves, you will be able to generate more force but no matter how hard you push, don't move.

### Neck Exercise #3: Resisted Protraction

With your fingers pointing upward, place the palms of your hands against your forehead. Press your head firmly forward against your hands. This is another isometric exercise. Balance your head above your shoulders and avoid any movement.

### Neck Exercise #4: The Side Press

With your fingers pointing upward, place the palm of your left hand against the left side of your head just above your ear. Press your head sideways against your hand. Hold for a slow count of five and then relax.

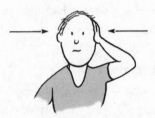

Now alternate using your right hand against the right side of your head. Hold for a slow count of five. Ten repetitions on each side is a reasonable target. Relax between each exertion.

This is another isometric exercise, so keep your head upright and balanced, and completely still.

## LEG AND BACK EXERCISES

### Leg Exercise #1: The Half Bend

Stand erect with your feet comfortably apart and your hands on your hips. Keep your feet flat on the floor. Slowly bend your knees. Just before you are halfway down, pause momentarily then straighten up again. Keep your back erect and your head balanced. Try not to tip forward.

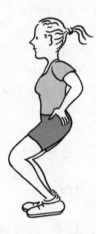

Move down and up slowly and smoothly. If you descend quickly, you are using gravity instead of your thigh muscles to lower your body. If you perform the exercise in a controlled fashion, you create a constant muscular tension that builds the strength you need.

### Leg Exercise #2: The Imaginary Chair

Stand with your back against a smooth wall. Place your feet slightly apart and about thirty centimetres (1 foot) in front of you. Let your arms hang at your sides. Press your back firmly against the wall and slide your body slowly downward until your thighs are parallel to the floor. Don't move your feet forward. Pressing your hands on the tops of your thighs is cheating; it takes the load off your thigh muscles. Your hands should hang free.

Stop when your hips and knees are each at a right angle and hold that position for as long as you can. When your legs have had enough of sitting on the imaginary chair, push yourself up again.

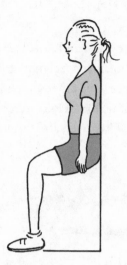

This exercise is an excellent way to build leg strength. You will discover that it is easier if you wear a coarse shirt and slide down a rough wall. To do it right, however, the wall should be smooth and you should slip down easily. If you can sit on the chair for thirty seconds, you're doing well. Start with a short time and gradually increase the duration as your endurance improves.

### Back Exercise #1: Arm Extension

This is a very gentle way to begin strengthening your paraspinal muscles. Lie face down with both arms straight out above your head. Raise one hand fifteen centimetres (six inches) off the floor and hold it there for a slow count of five. Slowly lower your arm. Don't let it fall. Pause for a moment then lift the other arm. You can start with ten repetitions but you should be able to increase the number fairly rapidly. Better yet, move to a more aggressive form of back strengthening.

Make the extension more taxing by lifting both arms together. Raising your arms this way requires your trunk muscles to steady your spine. Lifting both arms at once increases the amount of work the muscles must do.

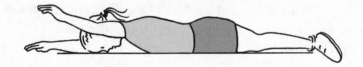

## Back Exercise #2: Hip Extension

Lie on your stomach and put your hands together under your forehead. You can turn your head to one side if you feel more comfortable that way. Bend one knee just enough to raise your foot. Now, holding that position, raise the front of your thigh off the floor. Hold your leg up for a slow count of five and then lower it again. Five to ten repetitions will probably be enough to start.

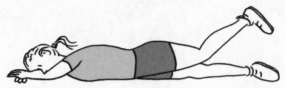

When you have finished one leg, repeat the exercise with the other. Rest between the repetitions.

The less you bend your knee, the more difficult the exercise becomes. To make it much tougher, lift both legs together.

The action of extending your hip requires the same muscular stabilization of your spine as when you lifted your arms. Because your legs weigh more, your back muscles work harder. Moving from arms to legs is a common progression in the exercise program.

## Back Exercise #3: Trunk Extension

Lie on your stomach with your hands clasped behind the small of your back. Tuck in your chin. Slowly raise your head and chest off the floor by arching your back. Hold your trunk elevated for a slow count of five and then gradually let yourself down. Keep breathing and rest between each repetition. Five to ten repetitions should be enough.

The exercise difficulty can be altered by changing the position of your arms. Holding your hands clasped behind the small of your back (Level 1) is the easiest. Holding your hands behind your neck with your fingers laced together and your elbows pointing out (Level 2) is more difficult. Holding your arms extended above your head with your elbows straight (Level 3) is the most difficult. Choose the level that is demanding but still allows you to perform the exercise correctly.

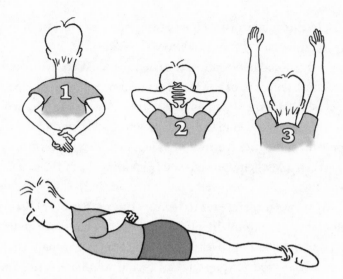

## Back Exercise #4: Trunk and Leg Extension

This exercise combines hip extension with trunk extension. You just do them at the same time. Begin lying on your stomach with your hands clasped behind the small of your back. Tuck your chin. Raise your head and upper body until your chest clears the floor. At the same time, bend your knees to raise your feet and then lift both thighs off the floor. This is a difficult exercise, and one that is never popular with someone suffering Pattern 2 pain.

You can make a tough exercise even tougher by changing your arm position from Level 1 to Level 2 or even Level 3. Want more? Try lifting your thighs up with your knees straight.

If you can manage all the difficult variations, the muscles in your buttocks and along your spine are in very good condition. It's time you used a Roman chair.

## Back Exercise #5: Isolated Lumbar Extension

I believe this exercise is one of the most important additions to our spine-exercise routines. Start by lying face down with your lower body on a flat surface. This may be the top of an exercise table, a bed, or, preferably, an inclined plane. The further you are tipped up, the easier the exercise becomes. In direct contrast to the sit-up, your feet must be anchored to prevent you from falling forward onto your head.

Your body should be unsupported from the waist up. With your hands clasped behind the small of your back, let your upper body droop forward. When you are hanging down as far as you can go, raise yourself slowly upward using the muscles in the small of your back. Concentrate on tightening only those muscles. Turning your legs in so that the toes on both feet are facing each other helps prevent you from using the muscles in your buttocks and thighs. Bring yourself up so that your back is straight and then sink slowly forward again. Five to ten repetitions may be all that you can manage to start. The number will increase as the endurance and strength in your back muscles improves. When you start, put a small stool on the floor below your head. If you feel the effort in your back is too much, use your arms to push up on the stool. The stool also helps you get positioned more easily.

For many people with chronic low back pain, starting this exercise is very uncomfortable. It should not reproduce your typical back pain, and any discomfort should subside rapidly once you are done. Don't let a short period of pain, no matter how unpleasant, discourage you from continuing. But if the exercise only reacquaints you with the symptoms you were hoping to forget, stop it. You can always try again later.

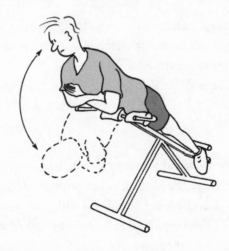

The exercise difficulty can be adjusted by altering the degree of incline; the steeper the incline, the easier the exercise. The standard piece of gym equipment, some variation of the Roman chair, is designed to be adjustable. You can also vary the difficulty by changing your arm positions. Level 1 is the easiest. The Level 2 position can be modified by holding your hands folded across your chest. Level 3, with your arms extended, is still the toughest. Want more? Use the Level 2 position with your arms over your chest and hold a free weight in your hands.

Because this exercise is initiated from a forward-flexed position, it is well tolerated by people with Pattern 2 pain. Surprisingly, it is also tolerated by Pattern 1 patients, despite the flexed posture, because gravity produces brief, intermittent traction when the trunk is hanging down, reducing the pressure on the discs. It is definitely worth a try.

### Back Exercise #6: The Sit-Down

This is the kindest way for many people to begin flexion exercises. Start by sitting on the floor hugging your knees. Keeping your feet on the floor and unanchored, hold onto your knees and gradually lean back as far as you can. When you have gone so far that you can no longer hold onto your knees, let your upper body sink to the floor.

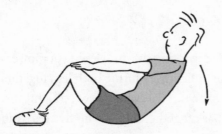

Push yourself back up with your arms. Grab your knees and do it again. The idea is to let your arms do most of the work and use your abdominal muscles to slow the descent of your upper body. The faster you fall backward, the less work they do. The more you can control the descent of your torso, the more your abdominal muscles benefit. Because it is a stretching exercise as well as an abdominal strengthening one, the sit-down is often recommended as the first back-flexion exercise.

### Back Exercise #7: The Leg Lift

Lie on your back and bend your left knee so that your left foot is flat on the floor beside your right thigh. Adopt a pelvic tilt by rolling your pelvis forward, tightening your buttocks and abdomen, and pushing the small of your back against the floor. Now without bending your right knee, lift your right leg up about fifteen centimetres (six inches) and hold it for a slow count of five. Lower it slowly, pause and do it again. Start with ten repetitions. When you have finished, straighten your left leg, bend your right knee and repeat the exercise on the other side.

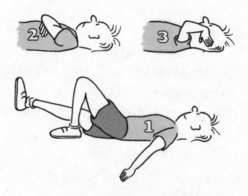

This is a gentle way of working the muscles in your lower abdomen. To make the exercise more difficult, try lifting both legs together. For variety, raise both legs in the air then, with your knees straight, spread your legs apart and bring them back together. Begin with five repetitions. If you lift both legs, be sure that you can maintain your pelvic tilt and keep your back flat on the floor. Arching your back may be uncomfortable but, more importantly, it allows your back muscles to help raise your legs, and diminishes the benefit to the lower abdominals.

The difficulty of single or double straight-leg raises can be increased by changing your arm position. The easiest version (Level 1) uses your arms as stabilizers. Put your arms on the floor and out to your sides. Keep your elbows straight and your palms down. Your hands should be about the level of your hips. They act like the big outriggers you see protruding from the sides of giant crane trucks.

Folding your arms across your chest (Level 2) makes the exercise more difficult. Placing your fingers behind your ears with your elbows bent and your arms on the floor (Level 3) is the most strenuous.

**Back Exercise #8: Crossover Knee Push**
Lie on your back with your knees bent and your feet flat on the floor. Adopt a pelvic tilt. Keep your back down, flex your left hip, and draw your left knee up toward your stomach. With your arm straight, place your right hand on your left knee. You will have to raise your head and shoulders. Be sure to keep your chin tucked in to lessen the strain on your neck. Now push your hand against your knee as hard as you can and feel the tension in your abdomen. Hold for a slow count of five and then lower your leg and your upper body. Pause and repeat. Ten repetitions is usual. When you have finished with your right arm and left knee, do the same thing with your left arm and right knee. This is a gentle introduction to abdominal strengthening exercises. It is supposed to be isometric, so avoid movement and concentrate on pitting one set of muscles against another.

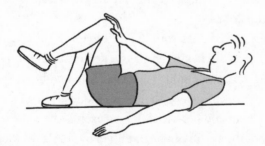

**Back Exercise #9: The Sit-up**
Lie on your back with your knees bent and your feet unrestrained and flat on the floor. Adopt a pelvic tilt. Hold your arms straight out in front of you above your knees and slowly raise your upper body until your shoulder blades clear the floor. Hold this elevated position for a slow count of five

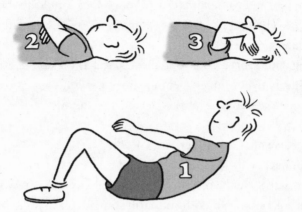

and then lower your upper body to the starting position. Five to ten repetitions is acceptable. Rest between each repetition. In spite of the many misconceptions that surround the sit-up, it is still a mainstay of any abdominal strengthening program. It is an excellent upper abdominal exercise.

As you begin, you may notice that you do not have sufficient strength to keep your feet flat on the floor. As you try to raise your upper body, your legs will lift as well. Lift your head and shoulders only as high as you can without lifting your feet. As your abdominal strength increases, your goal is to lift your upper body completely so that the lower points of your shoulder blades clear the floor.

Keep your chin tucked onto your chest. It helps to stare at a single spot over your head before you begin the sit-up. Keep your eyes on that spot as you lift up. Fixing your gaze holds your head still and helps prevents you from sticking out your chin. Poor sit-up technique is one of the commonest causes of neck pain and headache during exercise.

The difficulty of the sit-up can be modified by changing your arm positions. Holding your arms extended over your knees with your elbows straight (Level 1) is the easiest. Holding them folded across your chest (Level 2) makes the sit-up more difficult. Placing your fingers behind your ears and holding your elbows out to the sides (Level 3) is the most demanding arm position. I recommend fingers behind the ears instead of hands behind the neck since most people cheat by pulling their heads forward to help them sit up. That decreases the demand on the abdominal muscles. It is also an excellent way to produce Pattern 1 neck pain.

The ultimate sit-up is performed with the backs of your lower legs resting on a low bench or the seat of a chair. Keeping your hips and knees flexed and your feet unrestrained virtually eliminates muscular activity in your thighs and around your hips. In this position, your abdominal muscles must do all the work. The actual sit-up technique is exactly the same. Adopt a pelvic tilt and make sure that your head, neck, and shoulders come forward as a single unit. Stare at that spot on the ceiling. To make a difficult variation even harder, you can change your arm position from Level 1 to Level 3.

## Back Exercise #10: The Crunch

This exercise has become a popular substitute for the sit-up. The crunch or, as it should be done, the roll-up, includes elements of both a sit-up and a double leg lift. Done correctly, it is a very difficult exercise. It is seldom performed properly.

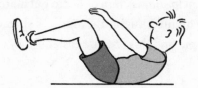

Lie on your back with both knees bent and your feet on the floor. Adopt a pelvic tilt. Tuck your chin in to avoid neck strain. Now fold your body up, bringing your head and shoulders forward the same way you do in a sit-up, and raising your legs with your knees bent in a double leg lift. Done properly, the crunch is a slow, steady movement that almost brings your chest to your knees. Once you have reached maximum flexion, slowly let go until you are back on the floor with your knees bent and your feet down.

You can make the crunch more difficult by changing your arm positions through the same three levels described for the sit-up. It is the rolling up that delivers the benefit and develops strength in both the upper and lower abdominal muscles. But usually when patients do crunches, they bob their heads, hunch their shoulders, and bounce their feet up and down on the floor. It is a generally pathetic effort that demands nothing of the abdominal muscles. Small wonder that so many patients tell me they have been doing crunches for months with no improvement. It depresses us both to find that, after all that time and effort, they still cannot perform a single unassisted sit-up. If you are going to do crunches, do them properly.

## Back Exercise #11: The Pelvic Thrust

This exercise is definitely not a pelvic tilt. It is a strenuous movement that exercises the lower abdominal muscles. Lie on your back with your knees bent and feet flat on the floor. Put your arms on the floor in the outrigger position used for Level 1 in Back Exercise #7, The Leg Lift. Now flex your hips and bend your knees until both are at a ninety-degree angle. Your thighs should be vertical and your lower legs should be parallel to the floor. Press down with your hands and raise your buttocks into the air. It sounds difficult, and it is. Don't bend your hips any more. This is not a roll-up. Your thighs should stay vertical and rise up when you lift your buttocks. If you have someone who can help you, ask him or her to put his or her arm in front of your thighs. When you lift straight up, your legs should not move your helper's arm. Most people find this exercise easier if they cross their ankles.

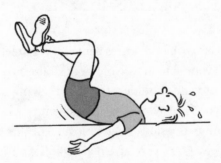

Try to hold the lift for a few moments before falling back. Five to ten repetitions will be quite enough to start. This exercise is so difficult that there is no arm progression. You need to push down with your arms in order to get the lift.

## Back Exercise #12: The Side Lift

The only muscles in the trunk that have not yet been exercised are the oblique muscles that wrap around the sides of your body. They run around your waist from their origins near the spine to their insertions into the fibrous layers that cover your abdomen. They are exercised when you bend to the side while standing or by performing an oblique sit-up or a side lift.

The technique for an oblique sit-up is the same as for an ordinary sit-up, but instead of coming straight forward, you come up on an angle aiming for the outside of your knee. Alternate the direction; sit up to your right and then to your left. It is a difficult exercise, and ten repetitions to each side is an accomplishment.

The most vigorous method of strengthening the muscles around your mid-section is a side lift. You may be able to use the same exercise table or sloping frame that you employed for Back Exercise #5: Isolated Lumbar Extension. This time, you lie on your left side with your feet secured and let your body drop sideways to the left. When you have reached the limit of your side bend, bring yourself back up into a straight line and then do it again. If you can manage ten repetitions, you are doing very well. When you are finished, rest for a moment then roll over and repeat the exercise, lying on your right side.

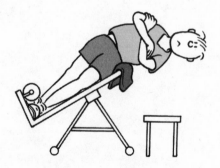

Having a small stool on the floor below your shoulder will let you use your lower arm to push yourself back up, if necessary. The higher the frame is tilted, the easier the side bend becomes. Working from a horizontal position, like the top of an exercise bench, is very difficult.

Both the oblique sit-up and the side lift can be made more challenging by changing your arm positions. The easiest position is with your arms folded across your chest. Raising them near your ears or extending them above your head makes it much tougher.

# CHAPTER SIXTEEN

## *On the Ball*

Over the past decade, North Americans have become acquainted with a new piece of fitness equipment, the exercise ball. Originally from Europe, the ball has become a hugely popular means of doing old-fashioned exercises in a new way. Exercise balls come in a variety of sizes; the sixty-five-centimetre-diameter ball is intended for a man of average height, the fifty-five-centimetre ball fits the average-sized woman.

Because the ball rolls freely, it is up to the user to provide the necessary stability. That stability is achieved in part by using the arm and leg muscles, but mainly by using the muscles in the abdomen and low back. Keeping yourself balanced on the ball promotes posture awareness that can translate into a better body position during normal daily activities.

Like any piece of equipment, the ball can magnify the benefits of your exercise. But it also has significant potential to aggravate your pain. The ball is not a substitute for your personal effort. For many exercises, it actually requires you to use more energy than performing the same exercise on a mat. Some patients seem to think that having a ball just means having fun. They think that the ball will do the job of exercising their spine. Just bouncing around on the ball brings little benefit. The ball is only a tool; you still have to do the work. For older patients and patients in poor physical condition, the extra effort may be too much.

Here are few of the many exercise-ball routines that you can try. The list is short, but it will give you an idea of how to start and what to expect.

### Ball Exercise #1: Sit On It

Sitting on the ball works muscles in the lower trunk and around the pelvis. Sit in a balanced position with your hands resting on your thighs. Keep your chest out and your shoulders down and back. Your feet should be on the ground. Stabilize your position by contracting your abdominal muscles and the muscles in your low back. Draw in your stomach, but keep breathing.

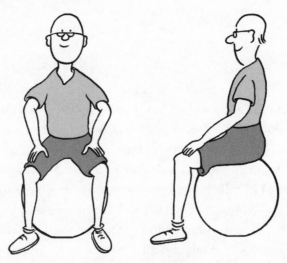

This sitting position is described as the neutral posture. For many of the remaining exercises, it is the correct starting point.

### Ball Exercise #2: How to Fall Off Your Ball

No matter how well you start, at some point you are bound to fall off. Don't fight the ball. Be calm and accept the fact that you are about to leave. Go with it and roll.

### Ball Exercise #3: The Pelvic Tilt

A pelvic tilt on the ball is no different than the pelvic tilt that you practised lying down. It is just more difficult to achieve. It works muscles in your lower abdomen, pelvis, and back. Tighten your stomach, roll your pelvis forward, and tense your buttocks. Try to maintain a straight upper back. To do the pelvic tilt on the ball, you must move out of the neutral posture.

### Ball Exercise #4: Legged Statue

Start in the neutral posture. Keep your chest out and your shoulders back. Tighten the muscles in your abdomen and low back. Now hold your arms straight out to the sides at shoulder height. Lift your left foot off the ground and extend your left knee. Hold your left leg straight out in front of you for a slow count of five and then put your foot down again. Lower your arms and relax. Now repeat the same exercise using your right leg.

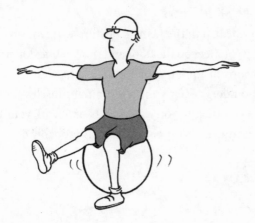

### Ball Exercise #5: Look Ma, No Feet

This exercise is a variation on Ball Exercise #4: Legged Statue. Start in the neutral posture then raise both arms out to the sides. Lift both feet off the ground and balance. If you can avoid touching your feet down for one minute, you are doing very well. Holding this position uses the muscles around your trunk and in your hips.

## Ball Exercise #6: Tough Tummy

To start this exercise, you lie face-down over the ball so that it presses up on your stomach. Both hands and both feet are on the ground. Keep your abdominal muscles tight and breathe normally. This is an isometric abdominal exercise. Try to keep the ball still. If it rolls away, you will have a chance to practise Ball Exercise #2: How to Fall Off Your Ball.

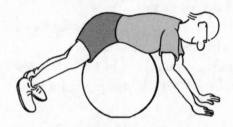

## Ball Exercise #7: Slide Down

Begin sitting on the ball in the neutral posture with your hands resting on your knees. Keep your feet on the floor and slowly slide down so that the ball gradually moves from under your buttocks, up your back, and finishes behind your shoulders. Keep your abdominal muscles tight, your knees bent, and your back straight. You will form an arch with your feet at one end and the ball at the other. A slow count of five is probably more than enough.

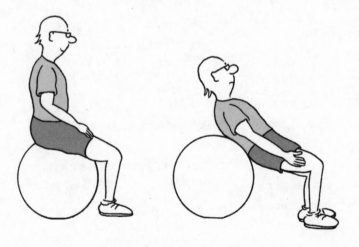

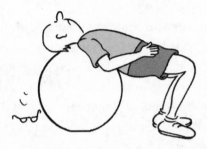

## Ball Exercise #8: The Bridge

In this exercise, you begin lying on your back on the floor with your feet resting up on the ball. Put your arms out to the side, palms up, with your hands at about waist level. Now slowly raise your hips until your body forms a straight line between your shoulders on the floor and your ankles (hopefully) still resting up on the ball. Use the muscles in your trunk, legs, and buttocks to keep the ball from rolling. Relax your shoulders.

If you master "The Bridge," you could progress to "The Swaying Bridge." Assume the bridge position, holding your body straight between your shoulders and your knees. Use the muscles in your trunk, buttocks, and abdomen to stabilize the ball and rock it from side to side in a slow, controlled movement. Don't let it roll away.

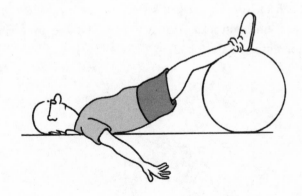

## Ball Exercise #9: Superman

Lie on the ball in the same position you used for Ball Exercise #6: Tough Tummy. Both your hands and feet are on the ground. Now lift your right leg and your left arm and hold them straight out. Tighten your abdominal muscles to prevent any side-to-side movement. Try to keep your back flat and level. Don't rotate your hips or lean to one side. Hold your right leg and your left arm up for a slow count of five and then put them down. Relax, then do it again using your left leg and your right arm.

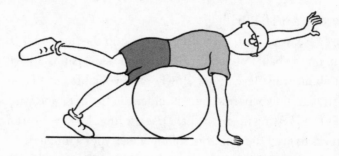

## Ball Exercise #10: Back Arches

For this exercise, you are lying on your stomach over the ball, but only your feet are on the ground. With your arms at shoulder level, reach down and grip the sides of the ball. Now arch your back. Slowly raise your head and shoulders up off the ball until your arms are out straight. Keep your pelvis on the ball and don't bend your knees. This exercise relies on muscles in your low back and buttocks. Your arms are used only for balance. It is the ball version of the Roman chair.

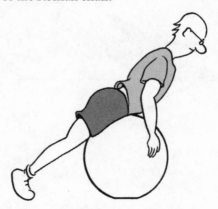

### Ball Exercise #11: Side Crunches

Doing side bends on an inclined plane is difficult. Doing them against the exercise ball is even harder. Lie on your left side with the ball at your waist. Cross your arms over your chest. Lift your upper body to the side until your trunk is perpendicular to the ball and your shoulders are parallel to the floor. Do not twist. You can wedge your feet at the bottom of a wall to help with balance. If you can manage it, this is an excellent exercise for those important side muscles that wrap around your midsection.

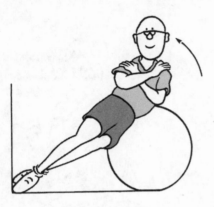

### Ball Exercise #12: Wall Squat

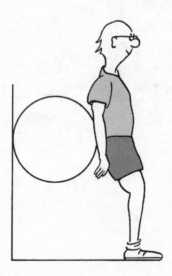
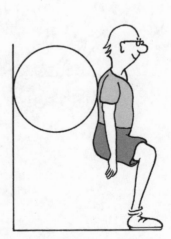

This exercise shows that you can use the ball to enhance almost any routine. Hold the ball behind you at waist height against a wall. Lean backward and trap it there. The ball should be pressing against your lower back. Now slowly bend your knees until you reach a sitting position. Keep your abdominal muscles tight and your back parallel to the wall. You are sitting on the imaginary chair from Leg Exercise #2 in Chapter 15, but the ball gets in the way.

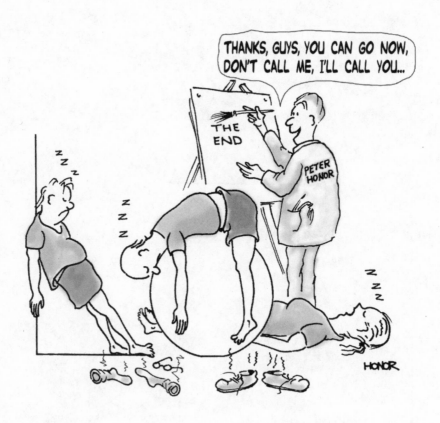

# INDEX

*Page numbers in italics indicate an illustration.*